# CELEBRITY Body ON A BUDGET

## CORNEL CHIN

PRICE WORLD
PUBLISHING

Prior to beginning any exercise program, you must consult with your physician. You must also consult your physician before increasing the intensity of your training.

Any application of the recommended material in this book is at the sole risk of the reader, and at the reader's discretion. Responsibility of any injuries or other adverse effects resulting from the application of any of the information provided within this book is expressly disclaimed.

---

Published by Price World Publishing, LLC
1300 W. Belmont Ave, Suite 20G
Chicago, IL 60657

---

Modeling by Dianne T. Goh and Matt Sulzer
Photos by Rob Price
Book cover, design and layout by Dianne T. Goh
Editing by Sherry Roberts
Printing by Sheridan Books, Inc.
Special thanks to Lifestyle Family Fitness in
Hilliard, Ohio for use of its facilities.

First Edition, March 2010
ISBN: 978-0-9724102-8-1
Library of Congress Control Number: 2009934041

Printed in the United States of America

10 9 8 7 6 5 4 3 2 1

# ACKNOWLEDGEMENTS

This book is dedicated to my parents Alonzo Tenlyn Chin and Florence Elenor Chin, who have influenced and shaped my life. I am eternally grateful for their 'Life' support and for providing myself and my brothers Ian and Darren with the most wonderful upbringing. We love you mum and dad.

I wish acknowledge the support, enthusiasm and commitment shown by my family and friends, particularly to my wife, Ania for her unconditional love and encouragement. I also seek forgiveness from my two little gems Rafal and Maksymilian for occasionally neglecting them during this writing process. I couldn't always get out with you on your bikes or play football and tennis with you! Daddy loves you always and will make it up to you- promise!

An extra special mention to Elizabeth Puttick for guiding me in the right direction in the vast world of publishing. Thanks for your expertise and steadfast dedication as my literary agent.

A mammoth thank you is in order to Andrew Prockter and David Arden and for your support, copy reading and especially for helping me when my computer didn't do what I wanted it to do. Thanks to Errol Arthur for his irritating phone calls each day-checking on me to make sure I was stuck to my desk working on this book.

Thanks and praise to the team at Price World Publishing, especially to Rob Price for giving me the opportunity to have my idea finally transformed into the 'Finished Article'

Finally, I would like to add a very special thanks to all of my clients for their understanding, support and for 'giving me time off' to write this book.

Thanks Barbara Maher for constantly asking me 'What's the latest on your book?' Your genuine interest is most appreciated, but I won't make your exercise sessions any easier!

For more fitness advice and information, Cornel's website can be visited at: **www.cmcfit.co.uk**

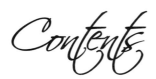

# Contents

## CHAPTER THREE:
## FIT YOUR BUDGET                                              51

## CHAPTER FOUR:
## ANALYZE THIS (PERSONAL FITNESS EVALUATION) 67

## CHAPTER FIVE:
## GYM, WHAT GYM? 89

# SOMETHING'S *gotta* GIVE

E ven in tough times, you can still shape up like a celebrity, even if you don't earn a celebrity's salary! With more than twenty years of experience in the field of fitness, I've shown Leonardo DiCaprio, Colin Firth, Audrey Tautou, Tilda Swinton, and many others how to do it, and I can show you. Incredibly, they've all achieved "film fitness" shape using my unique training methods, which require little exercise equipment.

> *"Cornel gave me the lean look I needed. His training methods are second to none!"* ~ **LEONARDO DICAPRIO**

This book can realistically provide you with the stepping stones to achieving that "drop dead gorgeous" celebrity body you've always admired and desired.

We're all trying to tighten our purse strings as the cost of living seems to be rising faster than the maximum speed of the treadmill at the gym. When the financial market is in turmoil or when the threat of escalating unemployment is present, your gym membership may seem like a luxury rather than a necessity. Don't get me wrong, gyms are a valuable environment in which to shape up. Most offer some of the most up-to-date, sophisticated equipment that will bend and shape you while you watch your favorite TV program. People are also attracted to the social side of being a club member, and many great relationships have been forged through this type of social interaction! So, if your pockets are still deep enough and you can continue to justify the cost of your gym membership, go and make use of it!

> *"Training with Cornel helped me achieve the good muscle tone and definition I needed for my film character."* ~ **AUDREY TAUTOU**

In poor financial climates, however, fitness clubs report declines in membership. Consumers are not so quick to flock to the hot new club that recently opened down the road. Existing club members, keeping a watchful eye on their monthly budget, often abandon their gyms. When times are tough, something's got to give.

As a gym member, you'll spend an average of 3 percent of your annual salary on the cost of your yearly membership. For some of you, this will be considered an investment in your overall well-being or even an absolute necessity. For others, a gym membership is just another high-cost luxury that gets pushed to the back of the line when considering monthly expenditures. But, exercise is more important than ever for staying healthy and is one of the best ways to keep positive and combat malaise in gloomy times.

If you're one of the many described above, you'll probably be pondering over these questions: What are my alternatives if I'm forced to cancel my membership through my job loss? How can I possibly stay fit and in shape without going to the club? I'm doing so well with my exercise program but simply can't afford to continue with my membership. I don't want to watch the rot set in! Help!

**"***I was no great fan of exercise until I met Cornel. He has given me a way of working out that is enjoyable, sustainable and effective. I'm enormously grateful to him for converting me.* **" ~ COLIN FIRTH**

So, for those of you who decided to save your hard-earned cash and not renew your gym membership, the good news is that you don't need a gym or expensive equipment to lose weight and get in shape. This book will show you the steps to getting fit and maintaining a great shape for significantly less than a month's membership at your gym.

*Celebrity Body on a Budget* unlocks the keys to low-cost or no-cost exercise solutions. You may think getting a good workout requires shelling out plenty of money for gym memberships or tons of equipment, but there are alternatives. This book will be your constant companion, providing exercise encouragement with useful solutions, tips, and practical ways for realistically achieving physical fitness success without stressing a dwindling bank account!

This book will change the way you think and feel about exercise. Gone are the days of over-complicated glitzy exercise machines that you never quite got the hang of and loud thumping, pumping music that deafened you when you were trying your hardest to fine-tune your body. *Celebrity Body on a Budget* is the definitive exercise manual to motivate and teach you that exercising on a budget is just as effective as going to the gym but a lot more fun and most certainly won't blow your budget. This book comes to your rescue by helping you achieve the kind of body you want through natural means and at an affordable price.

# CHAPTER *One:*

## KNOW THYSELF

# CHAPTER ONE:

## KNOW *thyself*

To get the best results out of something, you need to know how it works and what makes it tick. The same principle applies to your body. In fact, this applies even more so, since the human body is the most complex and sophisticated matter on this planet. The good news is that it doesn't take a science degree to grasp the rudiments of how your body best functions. In this chapter, I will take you through a step-by-step guide on body basics.

## BONES

Your skeleton provides the framework for the rest of your body. It supports the shape and form of your body in addition to protecting organs, allowing bodily movement, producing blood for your body, and storing minerals. The size and shape of your bones is genetically inherited, but it can also be influenced by what you eat and any disease you may encounter. You are born with about 300 to 350 bones; however, many bones fuse together between birth and maturity. As a result, an average adult skeleton consists of 208 bones.

Bones contain hard tissue that makes them both strong and durable. However, they are pliable and light enough to allow many types of movement requiring a lot of pressure without breaking. The basic chemical of bones is calcium phosphate. It's vital in your diet to keep your bones strong and healthy.

Your body's movement occurs at your joints. The amount of movement in your joints depends on the structure and function of the joint. The two basic types of joints for movement are the ball and socket joints (hips and shoulder joints) and hinge joints (elbow joint), which are usually limited to just a few movements.

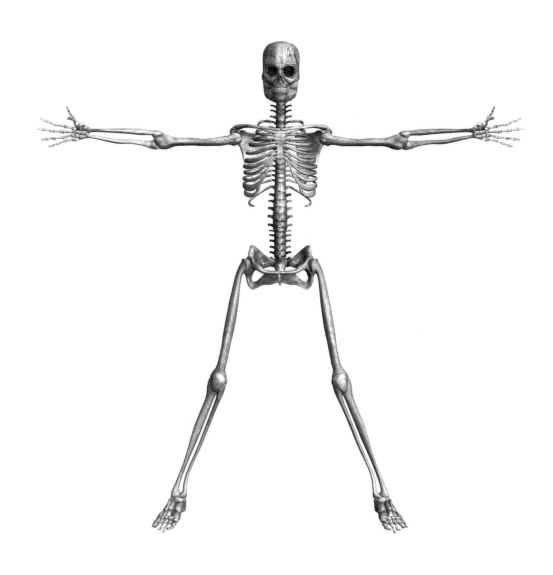

**Some joints have limited or no movement such as the bones of the skull. The ones that do permit free movement have three physical characteristics:**

1. Between the bones is a space called the synovial cavity. This contains synovial fluid, which helps to lubricate the action of the moving bones.

2. An articular cartilage covers the ends of the bones to keep them from rubbing directly on each other, while tough connective tissues called ligaments connect the bones to each other and provide stability to the joint.

3. Bones are attached to the muscles by tendons, which are fibrous cords of thick connective tissue.

**Your skeleton is highly important for five basic functions:**

1. Provides support for the soft tissues of your body to maintain an upright and erect posture.

2. Protects the vital internal organs of your body such as your brain, heart, and lungs.

3. Provides the framework for the attachment of muscles and serves as levers for your body's movement during muscular contraction.

4. Stores calcium and phosphorous, which make your bones sturdy and durable.

5. Contains chemical laboratories in the red marrow of the bones where red cells are produced. These carry oxygen to tissues of your body.

Male and female skeletons are similar but with a few slight differences. The bones of a male are slightly heavier and thicker, while women tend to have more shallow bones and a wider pelvis.

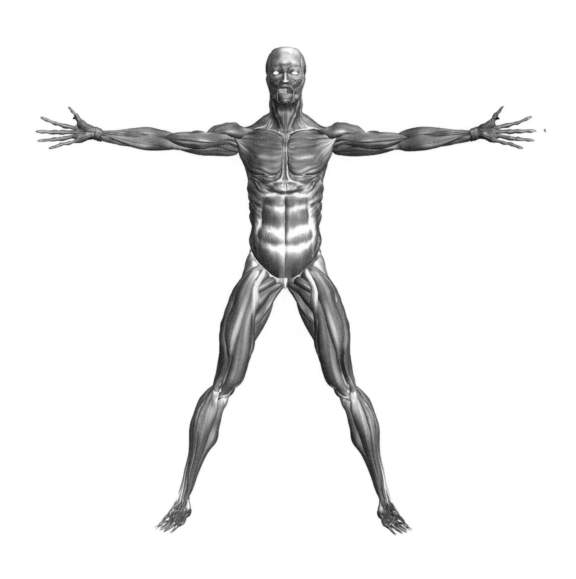

# I WANT MUSCLES

Your body houses three types of muscle tissue. These are smooth, cardiac, and skeletal and are characterized by location, microscopic structure, and nervous control. For the purpose of this book, you don't need to understand the intricacies of the entire muscular system. Muscles are attached to bones and contain the contractile elements necessary to produce movement.

A muscle is a collection of cells called muscle fibers that lie next to one another and may vary in size from a fraction of an inch to in excess of a foot in length. Each muscle fiber is encapsulated in a sheath of connective tissue. Groups of muscle fibers are bound together to form a bundle of muscle tissue called fasciculus, and these, in turn, are wrapped in additional bundles of connective tissue to form muscle itself. The connective tissue that surrounds the various bundles of the muscle fibers attaches to the end to form a muscle tendon. It's estimated that there are 250 million muscle fibers in your body. There are approximately 650 voluntary muscles (muscles which you have control of). Skeletal muscles account for about 45 percent of the body weight of a man and about 36 percent in women.

## The basic function of the muscular system is to:

**1.** Work with your skeletal system to produce movement.

**2.** Allow your body to maintain posture.

**3.** Aid in heat production.

An obvious movement of the body is walking, which involves the action of many muscles. The movement of a body part, such as flexion of the forearm at the elbow joint, results from contraction of the bicep muscle (front upper arm) and relaxation of the tricep muscle (rear upper arm). Contraction of skeletal muscles holds the body in a stationary position. Without such contractions, your body would collapse to the ground. Muscular contractions also produce heat by their movements and play an important role in maintaining body temperature.

## ENERGIZE ME!

Without food, your body will run out of energy—food is your fuel. Therefore, food provides your ultimate stores of energy. The various foods you consume are, over time, broken down into various energy blocks.

Once the food is broken down, your greatest energy fuel is called adenosine triphosphate (ATP). Some of this is stored in your muscles ready for immediate explosive action. This is generally available for emergency situations, but also for when you require the most powerful effort in your activity. Unfortunately, there are limited amounts of ATP for the first few seconds of really dynamic activity, such as a quick dash to catch a bus.

Your body also possesses another fuel source that can be converted into ATP. This is known as PCr (creatine phosphate). It takes a little longer to "kick in," and so the energy production is slightly less explosive. PCr enables you to continue fairly explosive effort for about twenty seconds.

For longer term muscle fuel, the body uses glycogen (glucose derivation). It is less explosive than ATP but is longer lasting. This type of energy supply lasts up to forty seconds and is readily available in your muscles.

For lower level, longer term activity, you can also utilize fat as your main source of fuel. For fat to be drawn on as your body's fuel source, it is widely known that you need to exercise at approximately 60 to 70 percent of your maximum intensity.

Although the systems using these various types of human energy fuel don't operate entirely independently of each other, you can see where the main energy source will be for different types of activities. As an example, long-distance runners focus mainly on training the aerobic system, while a javelin thrower will require more short-term energy in the form of ATP.

## WHAT'S MY TYPE?

This section shows you how to identify your body type and shape, as well as how to make the most of it through exercise.

Depending upon your genetics, as well as your exercise and eating habits, your body shape may be quite different from those around you. Some body types make us appear like human waste disposals, while others suggest the equivalent of a human fat magnet. No two bodies are the same, and that's why what works for one of your friends may not necessarily work as well for you. Your body's blueprint was determined on the day you were born.

Although you may dislike the body type or shape that you were born with, you can't change your basic body form, and it sets natural limits to what you can achieve. But don't get discouraged! There are ways to make the most of what you have. You can change your body composition (fat to muscle ratio) and firm up untoned areas with exercise and healthy eating. It is possible to redesign and make the most of what Mother Nature gave you. Whatever your body type, this book will help to bring out the best in your body.

Your body shape will generally fall into one of three main categories: ectomorph, mesomorph, and endomorph. However, most of us tend to be a combination of these, as few people actually fall distinctly into one category. Common combinations include ecto-mesomorph and endo-mesomorph.

# MEE! ECTOMORPH, ENDOMORPH AND MESOMORPH

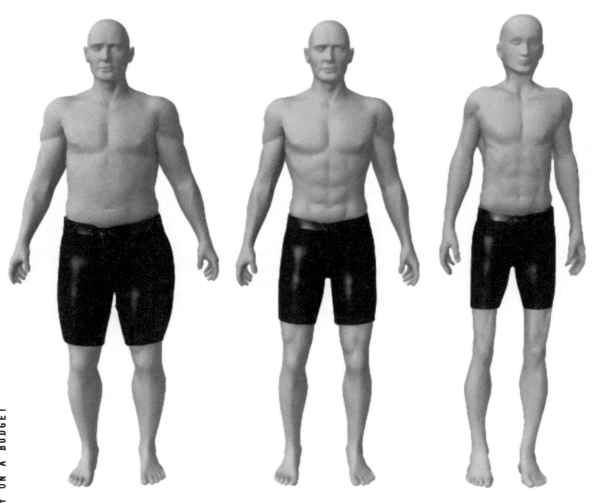

## ECTOMORPHS:

They are characterized by having long torsos and slim hips and shoulders. They generally have delicate bone structures in proportion to their height and are good at physical activity. Ectomorphs can lose weight easily and are inclined to low levels of body fat; they struggle to put on weight and muscle.

### Cardio training strategy:

Your goal is to up your stamina and whip your heart and lungs into shape, but simultaneously add muscle mass, so limit your cardio exercise to no more than three times a week. Aim for twenty to forty minutes per session at a moderate workout level.

### Resistance training strategy:

Build up muscle with two to four sets of resistance training exercises per body part. Use a moderate-to-heavy weight that you can lift with good form for six to ten repetitions. As you improve, consider doing a split routine, in which you work some parts of the body one day and then others the next.

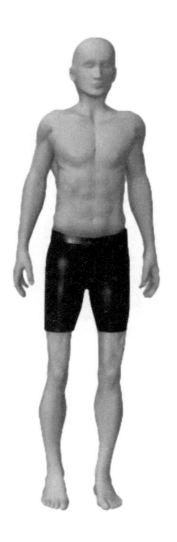

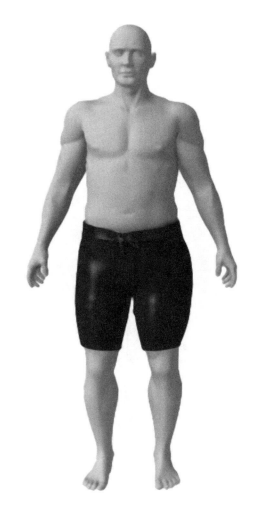

### ENDOMORPHS:

Endomorphs tend to have bigger bones than the other body types. They usually have round faces with larger thighs and hips. Endomorphs often have arms and legs that are short and tapered, giving them a stocky appearance. Most endomorphs have comparatively small hands and feet and a high waist. Although endomorphs have higher levels of body fat than the other body types, they can also build muscle and lean mass fairly easily. Weight loss is most difficult for the endomorph body type.

**Cardio training strategy:**
Focus on doing thirty to sixty minutes of cardio work three to six times a week for maximum fat and calorie burn. Your cardio workouts should generally be done at a moderately intense level.

**Resistance training strategy:**
Emphasize your curves by adding muscle tone. Perform a total-body weight training routine three times a week, on nonconsecutive days, that consists of two sets of weight training exercises per body part. Do ten to fifteen repetitions per set using a moderate-to-light weight. To improve body symmetry, you may want to increase the amount of upper body exercises. Try an extra set of exercises.

## MESOMORPHS:

They possess the ideal body shape and are usually described as having a more robust and athletic build. They tend to have an hourglass or ruler shape, and gain muscle mass easily. The majority of mesomorphs have broad shoulders and a narrow waist. They have a fast metabolism and can lose weight more easily than endomorphs.

### Cardio training strategy:

Aiming for three to five cardio workouts a week done at a moderate-to-fast pace should help keep you looking lean and trim. Aim for thirty to forty-five minutes per session.

### Resistance training strategy:

Utilizing light-to-moderate weight training done two to three times a week will help enhance tone, not size. You should complete a basic strength training workout twice a week, performing two sets of twelve to fifteen repetitions using light-to-moderate weights for each major muscle group. The circuits in this book (moving quickly from one exercise to the next without a break) are ideal, as they will promote strength and stamina without building too much bulk.

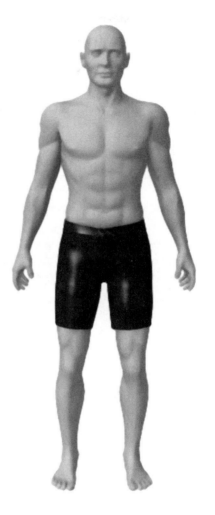

To draw a conclusion, remember that no one body type is better or worse than another. Whatever your body shape, the best body shape is the one you were born with based on your genetic makeup. How you wear it is up to you. Any body type can be healthy and fit and look great! You should realize and learn to accept that not all women are meant to be fashion model size and all men are not meant to be as well defined as the cover models in the latest men's fitness magazines. While you cannot change from one body type to another, you can improve your shape and make the best of your body. After all, your body size and structure reflect not only your genetics, but also your eating and exercise habits. You are who you are, and no one else can be you!

## FITNESS FUNDAMENTALS

Exercise is to your body what fine-tuning is to the engine of your car.
It enables you to perform up to your potential. Fitness can be described as a
condition that helps you look, feel, and do your best.

More specifically, it is the ability to perform daily tasks vigorously and
alertly, with energy left over for enjoying leisure time activities and meeting
emergency demands. It's the ability to endure, bear up, withstand stress, and
carry on in circumstances where an unfit person could not continue; in short,
physical fitness is a major basis for good health and well-being.

Fitness involves the performance of your heart, lungs, and muscles. Also, since
what you do with your body also affects what you can do with your mind,
fitness influences, to some degree, qualities such as mental alertness and
emotional stability.

As you took the first step by purchasing this book, it's important to remember
that fitness is an individual quality that varies from person to person. It's
influenced by age, gender, heredity, personal habits, exercise,
and eating habits.

## FREQUENTLY ASKED QUESTIONS:

### FACT 1:

*How much can I change my body shape—could
I, an endomorph, ever look like an ectomorph
with the right training?*

Your genetic inheritance and your environment both hold strong
influences on your body shape and size. Remember, your body
is not infinitely malleable! If your parents are short and stocky,
you can achieve good muscle definition and reduce excess
weight, but you may never make the cover of a glossy magazine.
Similarly, if you are tall and thin, you may never be able to "bulk
up" like a female shot putter. You may increase your muscle size,
improve your muscular definition, and decrease body fat, but you
may struggle to become an Olympic athlete.

# BACK TO BASICS

**Fitness is most easily understood by examining its four components:**

## 1. CARDIO-RESPIRATORY ENDURANCE:

the ability to deliver oxygen and nutrients to tissues and to remove wastes, over sustained periods of time. Long runs and swims are among the methods used in measuring this component.

## 2. MUSCULAR STRENGTH:

the ability of your muscles to exert force for a brief period of time. Upper body strength, for example, can be measured by various weightlifting exercises.

## 3. MUSCULAR ENDURANCE:

the ability of your muscle, or a group of muscles, to sustain repeated contractions or to continue applying force against a fixed object. Push-ups are often used to test endurance of chest, arm, and shoulder muscles.

## 4. FLEXIBILITY:

the ability to move your joints and use muscles through their full range of motion. The sit-and-reach test is a good measure of flexibility of the lower back and the backs of the upper legs.

## FACT 2:

*How much of a role does genetics play in how I look?*

The basic shape of your body is actually preset from birth. Everybody is born with a different body type. This is why everyone has a different body shape and develops different levels of body fat and muscle mass. Your body type is completely determined by genetics. You will probably share the same body type as one of your parents, or your sister or brother. Because body type is a genetic trait, it is usually difficult or impossible to change body types.

# THE HEART OF THE MATTER —
# HOW TO MEASURE YOUR HEART RATE

Using your own heart rate is an excellent method for measuring intensity during cardiovascular activities. Exercise that doesn't raise your heart rate to a certain level and keep it there for twenty minutes won't contribute significantly to cardiovascular fitness.

To maximize the benefits of exercising, it is important to exercise at the right intensity. This intensity level can be determined by using your heart rate as a guide. For effective aerobic exercise, your heart rate should ideally be maintained at a level between 65 and 85 percent of your maximum heart rate as you exercise. The heart rate you should maintain is called your target heart rate or training zone. This varies with your physical condition and your age.

You can find your training zone in the chart below. Training zones are listed for both unconditioned (**Exercise Neophyte and Progressive Exerciser**) and conditioned (**Adventurous Exerciser and Specialist Exerciser**) according to age.

| Age | Conditioned Training Zone (beats per minute) | Unconditioned Training Zone (beats per minute) |
|---|---|---|
| 20 | 138-167 | 133-162 |
| 25 | 136-166 | 132-160 |
| 30 | 135-164 | 130-158 |
| 35 | 134-162 | 129-156 |
| 40 | 132-161 | 127-155 |
| 45 | 131-159 | 125-153 |
| 50 | 129-156 | 124-150 |
| 55 | 127-155 | 122-149 |
| 60 | 126-153 | 121-147 |
| 65 | 125-151 | 119-145 |
| 70 | 123-150 | 118-144 |

## CHECKING YOUR HEART RATE

### STEP 1
Check your pulse at your wrist, not the neck. Studies have shown that applying pressure to the carotid artery in the neck can slow your heartbeat, causing you to miscalculate.

### STEP 2
Use two fingers—your index and middle—not your thumb. The thumb has a pulse of its own and can interfere with an accurate count.

### STEP 3
Count to ten and multiply that number by six to get your heart rate. This is a compromise between counting for six seconds (too quick and possibly less accurate) and counting for fifteen seconds, by which time the heart rate slows.

### STEP 4
Practice finding your pulse so you can begin counting immediately. If it takes twenty to thirty seconds to find your pulse, your heart rate will have significantly slowed.

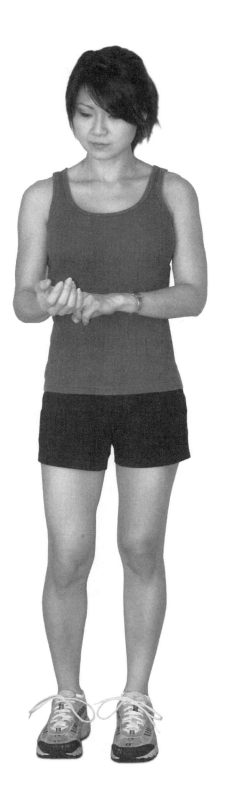

# CHAPTER
## *Two:*
## LET'S GO ALTERNATIVE

# LET'S GO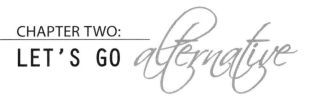

## HOW TO 'SNEAK' EXERCISE INTO YOUR EVERYDAY LIFE

With work and life balance, it can often feel that there is hardly any time to relax, let alone exercise. However, among all of these daily activities lay opportunities for simple activities that burn calories and can go a long way to helping in your weight loss quest. You'll soon discover that once you develop the habit of performing some or all of the simple tips highlighted in this chapter, you will gain important tools for your fitness campaign and might not even notice that you're exercising throughout the day!

Whether you're at work or out and about shopping, these great activities can really go a long way in helping you stay in shape and stave off excess calories. In this chapter, you'll be encouraged to be, and stay, as generally active as possible. If done regularly, you'll soon realize that with the help of this book, fitness and weight loss really can be achieved by adapting simple changes to your lifestyle when doing household chores or performing other minor tasks.

### FIND A DIFFERENT ENTRANCE.

When visiting the shopping center, park your car near the entrance farthest from your destination. You can then walk the added distance to the store or department you want to visit. During the summer, this can be a great way to rack up plenty of steps inside a comfortable, air-conditioned space.

### PUT DOWN THE REMOTE.

Whenever you watch TV or listen to music at home, leave the remotes on the shelf and control everything by hand. By forcing yourself to stand up and walk a few steps each time you change the channel or adjust the volume, you can build in important bursts of movement into your most sedentary activities.

## WALK IN; DON'T DRIVE-IN.

When eating on the go, resist the urge to use the drive-in window. Instead, park your car and walk into the restaurant to place your order. Without too much trouble, you could add one hundred steps to your daily tally. Furthermore, as most people stay in their cars and clog the drive-in queue when getting a quick bite, you might not lose any time at all by walking inside. You'll also make a small saving on fuel too as you won't be idling your car engine while you're stuck in the drive-in line.

## WASH THE CAR.

When it's time to wash the car, do it yourself instead of driving through the overpriced automatic car wash. Initially, you may want to try pay-as-you-go car washes, which allow you to use equipment similar to the automatic systems but also encourage you to walk around the car and stretch your muscles. If you want to devote more time to washing your car, you can buy the necessary products and work from home. In either case, you'll benefit from both the financial savings and by adding exercises into your routine. You'll probably clean your car better than the automated systems ever could.

## FLEX YOUR MUSCLES WHEN SITTING DOWN.

Whether you're relaxing at home or sitting behind your desk at work, there are a number of simple exercises you can perform without standing up. When seated, try to flex and release both your abdominal and gluteus/buttock muscles. Even when you don't have a chance to move, squeeze in these isotonic exercises to help along your fitness regimen.

## STRETCH YOUR FREE TIME.

If you have a little more space to stretch your muscles, devote some time to simple movements that can improve your flexibility. Whether you choose to stretch your arms, legs, or entire body, simple stretching movements are the perfect addition to relaxing moments.

## MOVE WITH THE PHONE.

When on the phone at home or at work, try to pace up and down or do a short series of exercises such as calf raises and squats. If you're using a mobile phone or a cordless handset, you shouldn't have any trouble taking a few steps back and forth. Walk up and down the stairs to burn more calories. If using a corded handset, try marching on the spot with your knees high.

## YOUR HOUSEHOLD CHORES WORKOUT

Between never-ending household projects and picking up after the day's various activities, there doesn't seem to be much time left for taking care of yourself. But a hectic schedule is still no reason to forgo your daily workout. So, what solutions are out there if you find yourself housebound and always pressed for time, but keen to exercise?

Look no further than your broom closet for a workout. Household chores to keep in shape may not seem like the most obvious solution to fitness, but it is one that has numerous benefits. Digging into household chores can be a great way to burn calories and tone up your muscles.

You may think to yourself, "Surely, vacuuming the stairs or doing laundry isn't going to help me lose weight and tone muscles!" Once you have actually convinced yourself to start household chores, the advantages flow in for everyone, not just the family member on whose shoulders the chores normally fall.

The benefits of sneaking in some extra calorie-burning chores are enormous. With a little creativity, you can make exercise a part of your routine no matter how long your to-do list is. Since just thirty minutes of housework a day rates as light exercise, there really is an amazing way to incorporate exercise into your daily routine.

# TOP 10
## HOUSEHOLD CHORES FOR BURNING CALORIES

(Calorie expenditure estimations are based on a 150-pound person and 60 minutes of activity)

### CHORE/ACTIVITY CALORIES

| | CHORE/ACTIVITY | CALORIES |
|---|---|---|
| 1. | Moving furniture | 450 |
| 2. | Scrubbing floors | 380 |
| 3. | Raking leaves | 342 |
| 4. | Gardening | 324 |
| 5. | Mowing the lawn | 324 |
| 6. | Washing the car | 306 |
| 7. | Cleaning windows | 310 |
| 8. | Vacuuming | 168 |
| 9. | Washing dishes | 152 |
| 10. | Doing laundry | 144 |

Housework utilizes all of your muscle groups. This, in turn, builds endurance, tone, strength, and suppleness. For example, picking up the children's toys works the muscles in your arms and shoulders. Hauling those toys throughout the house also works your legs and buttocks. Walk the length of your house while vacuuming, and you will enjoy a full body workout that will also burn calories and increase your heart rate if you vacuum at a fast pace.

Take a look at the chart above to get an idea of how effective chores can be at eating up those unwanted calories.

# WHAT CLASSIFIES HOUSEHOLD CHORES AS EXERCISE?

Keeping fit should be fun, but it should also fit in with your life because it's not always possible to find time for a jog or a bicycle ride. Fitting household chores into your fitness schedule is a perfect compromise.

All chores can be exercise in some form or other because they generate activity. However, it's reasonable to state that some chores are more beneficial for you than others. For example, vacuuming your entire house is obviously more strenuous than, say, loading your washing machine.

Dusting can also be good exercise, but that is not to say that all chores where you stand still are not as good for you as those where you move. Ironing, in particular, is supposedly very good, and half an hour of ironing counts toward your exercise for the day.

**Here are some moves to help you step up the normal pace of your usual housework and to show you how to work in ways to get in some aerobic moves and toning exercises. You could have a total body workout on your hands!**

## 1. MOP 'TILL YOU DROP.

Using a bucket and mop requires more work, lifting and carrying the bucket, wringing out the mop, possibly mopping the area twice—once with detergent and once with clean water—which all add to calories burned. Besides greatly multiplying the workload and working your arms, chest, hips, and back muscles, your floor will be sparkling!

## 2. WAX TO THE MAX.

Next time you want a major workout and the paint job on your car is looking dull, don't put it off—waxing your car for an hour and a half will burn off a mega-amount of calories. All that bending, twisting, and moving up and down the body of the car is great for overall flexibility. Adding pressure to your wax job with your hands works your shoulder muscles and helps prevent "bingo swingers" (those floppy backs of arms).

### 3. SUCK IT UP.

Vacuuming is great exercise, especially if you make a conscious effort to concentrate on contracting your chest and muscles at the back of the arms as you push out and then focusing on your upper back and biceps as you pull the vacuum cleaner backwards. By using the brush option on a carpeted surface, you will add additional resistance to your workout, burning more calories per push! Be sure to change sides to encourage balance in your effort.

### 4. WEED IT AND REAP.

Weeding for an hour will have you sweating and puffing. Adopt the all-fours position using a pad under your knees for comfort and start pulling and tugging at the weeds. This activity conditions the muscles in your stomach, upper and lower back, shoulders, forearms, and biceps.

### 5. SQUEAKY CLEAN.

Washing your mirrors and windows makes for great stretching and toning exercises. The combination of up and down movements will work wonders for your legs, buttocks, and shoulder muscle groups. While performing these up and down movements, try incorporating the "squat," which is one of the greatest exercises for your thigh and buttock muscles. It's simple! Place your feet hip-width apart. As you move downwards, simply bend at your knees to lower the buttocks to approximately a right angle; as you move upwards, extend your legs to return to the start position. To engage the shoulders, add a little pressure against the surface of the area to be cleaned for increased toning. Take care not to push against the mirror or windows too hard (crack!) and change hands occasionally.

### 6. GET ORGANIZED.

Been putting off that major reorganizing or cleaning out project for ages? Classify it as exercise and get it done! Why not take the contents of your cupboards, bookshelves, wardrobes, etc. out, then reach up and put them back in, in an orderly and organized way? You're getting in another great upper body workout! The reaching and lifting are great for increasing the suppleness and tone to the shoulders, arms, and back muscles. Stepping up on a secure step ladder for reaching those high shelves is a big bonus for the legs and buttocks.

### 7. STEP TO IT.

While wiping down your banister and handrails, substitute your step class, by using the steps in your house. As you wash and wipe down, try to vary the moves: First, step up and down on the bottom step for two to three minutes; rest a minute or two and repeat. As an additional approach: holding onto the handrail, walk up and down the first three stairs (great for butts and thighs). When you get the hang of that, try walking briskly up and down the stairs a few times (use the handrail for support).

### 8. DON'T TAKE IT EASY.

Resist the urge to take your everyday household at a slow pace—instead increase your heart rate by doing exercises such as squats, push-ups, and abdominal crunches in between tasks. Make an extra couple of trips up the stairs while carrying the vacuum cleaner or do a set of push-ups when switching the laundry from the washer to the dryer. Why not shape up your calves while brushing your teeth or combing your hair? How about stretching your legs while the kettle's boiling? It's so simple to add in exercises at almost every opportunity.

## SEVEN BEST HOUSE CHORES TIPS

1. Think safety first—take care lifting heavy buckets, etc. Be aware of slippery surfaces and bend your knees when picking up items from the floor.

2. For motivation, plan your household chores schedule and stick to it. Put it in your diary as an actual appointment and stick to that date.

3. If you need to take several items up or down the stairs, then take them one at a time. So it takes longer, but you'll burn more calories, and your legs will love you for it.

4. Hide your remote controls for the TV, video, or stereo system. To switch channels, rely on good old leg power instead. If you did this ten times daily, you'd be surprised to learn that you could burn off the equivalent of a large croissant over four weeks.

5. Each week build up your time or add in more activities for ongoing improvement.

6. If you can't fit it all in, in one hit, try dividing your chores over the course of the day—ten minutes of laundry in the morning, followed later by vacuuming for another ten minutes, and in the evening perhaps mopping.

**7.** Add intensity. The key to turning any household task into exercise is to pick up the pace or intensity and sustain it for as long as comfortably possible without resting. For example, if you have three floors to mop, throw on some headphones with upbeat music, put some major muscle behind your scrubbing, and time yourself to see if you can get a sparkling result under a certain time limit. This will help you keep the activity intense enough that it counts as exercise.

Finally, while doing housework may not appeal to everyone as the ideal mode of fitness, on those days when you need to cross-train but are short on time, it might offer the perfect solution to your dilemma. Furthermore, you'll end up with a gleaming kitchen, sparkling furniture, neatly folded clothes, and a dust-free house. What better way to get fit and burn undesired calories?

## USE EXERCISE WHILE COMMUTING

### DON'T LET THE TRAIN TAKE THE STRAIN

Okay, so you've got a stressful job and a demanding lifestyle and realistically can't always spare the time to exercise an hour each day. For starters, that's the wrong attitude! If you commute to work every day, you have the perfect chance to slip in some outdoor exercise.

The hassle of commuting to and from work eventually takes its toll on you, especially the impact it can have on your health. All that time in the car or train can negatively affect you not just physically, but mentally. Moving closer to work is an expensive option, considering the associated costs, and looking for a new job in these financially hard times is probably not a practical idea either. The good news is that you can find ways to get exercise while commuting, improving your health and making you feel better.

There are few things worse for your body than a long commute and a sedentary desk job. Your body and mind need a chance every day to burn excess energy, or you're likely to begin storing it in the form of love handles and a barrel for a stomach.

It's a known fact that people who build exercise into their working day have more energy, are calmer, are better at problem solving, and find it easier to concentrate than on days when they don't exercise. Also, being active will make you feel much more productive. So, a little variety in your commute could go a long way to improving your day in the office. Is there a better way to start the day than by combating climate change, preventing obesity, and saving a little money, all on your way to work?

**No matter what form of transportation you take, there are exercises you can do. Carry a bottle of water with you and wear appropriate loose clothing. You can change when you get to work. Here are some of the best commuting exercise ideas:**

1. Be an early riser. Before you consider how you're going to get to work, get out and go for a twenty- to thirty-minute jog, bike ride, or swim. You have the most energy in the morning, and you can feel good knowing that you've done more before 7:00 a.m. than most people will do all day. If you can, do this with your partner or a friend who will keep you motivated.

2. Not only are bikes and legs recession-busting forms of transportation, but by throwing exercise into the mix, you kill the commuting and fitness birds with one stone! Combining exercise with something you have to do anyway—getting to work—means you're more likely to keep it up. Walk or take a bike to work whenever possible. Cycle all or part way, then take public transportation the rest of the trip into work. You get the benefit of a ride in the morning and again on the return trip home, and you're helping to save the planet and save money by leaving the car resting comfortably in the garage.

3. In the mornings, if you really must commute by car, get to work a few minutes early so you have time for a longer walk from the parking garage. When you arrive, park as far away as possible from your place of work and briskly walk the rest. If you take the farthest parking space, the extra walk will rack up those all important steps. You also may have an easier exit at the end of the day as well. If you can't park further away, then walk around the building twice before heading into the office.

4. If traveling by subway/metro/train, find out how far it is to the bus or train station from your home and office. You can use this trip for exercise by jogging or power walking to the bus or train.

   Employ brisk walking between station or platform changes. Take the stairs more frequently or whenever possible instead of escalators or lifts; use your legs with each step by taking two steps at a time. Stand whenever you're traveling, hold the handrail with one hand, and slightly lift a foot off the floor. Switch arms and feet with each station stop. You'll challenge your core balancing muscles, legs, and arms.

5. When taking the bus, get off a stop or two earlier or after your usual stop, briskly walk the rest of the way.

6. Keep it interesting. Nothing is less motivating than a workout that feels like work. No sense being a slave to your commute to work. Try different walking, cycling, or running routes, or set a goal that you can work toward. For example, try shaving off a few minutes each week by walking faster. Keep note of your previous week's times.

# HIT THE ROAD

Spending a lot of time in a car while commuting to and from work or on any road trip can have a negative impact on your health and muscle tone. As a commuter, you might drive for twenty minutes to the local rail station and spend up to five minutes searching for a place to park before walking to the station. Driving simply isn't a healthy activity—whether it's the stress and frustration of dealing with traffic or the very real risk of being involved in an accident.

The ideal thing would be to eliminate the hour-long round trip commute. That's a lot of time to be cooped up, and if it's a driving commute, it's going to take a toll on your health in one form or another.

**When a car journey is your only option, you can arrive at your destination refreshed and toned by doing some isometric (static) exercises when stuck in traffic jams. Just be careful and pay attention to your driving and traffic. Apply your handbrake when necessary and be fully aware of your actions and surroundings. There aren't many health benefits to a car accident! Try these for size:**

## 1. TUMMY TONER:

Sit up straight in the seat in a normal driving position. Breathe in deeply into your lower abdomen. Now instead of exhaling, push the air up to your chest, filling your upper lungs. Now slowly exhale. You will feel your posture improve and get a big rush of energy by doing this exercise. You may need to readjust your mirrors due to a higher seating position.

## 2. STEERING WHEEL ISOMETRICS:

Grasp the wheel firmly in both hands. Push in like you are trying to crush the wheel. Now lean forward and pull out like you're trying to stretch the wheel. These exercises will help firm the chest and upper arm muscles.

## 3. TUMMY SUCKER:

Inhale normally, lean forward a bit, exhale normally but right at the end blow out just a little more very quickly. Then sit up before the next inhale. As an alternate, try sitting up while making the extra exhale.

## 4. STEERING WHEEL ISOMETRIC CURLS:

Grasp the wheel with both hands, lean forward, and pull up toward you. Don't pull too hard, as it is easy to damage the steering shaft this way. Just pull enough to flex your biceps and shoulders.

### 5. STRESS BUSTER:

If you are getting tired or stressed, try tapping your head. Use the fingertips of one hand to tap your head just above the hairline while you steer with the other hand. Tap firmly but not painfully. The object is to stimulate the blood flow in the scalp. Tap while saying to yourself, "I release this stress, and I choose to relax and be happy in this moment."

### 6. EYE TO EYE:

Nothing gets more stress while driving than your eyes. Blink often to keep them wet. Move them around while driving instead of staring straight ahead. Use a pattern like ahead, mirror, ahead, instruments, ahead, left, ahead, right, ahead, mirror, etc. When rubbing the eyes, start by placing your index and middle fingers on the bridge of your nose. With firm and steady pressure, move outward along the eyebrow and then down the cheekbone. Follow the cheekbone around to the nose and back up to the bridge. Never reverse the circle, as it will cause the tender skin under the eye to get stretched and look baggy.

### 7. WIGGLING IT JUST A LITTLE BIT:

While seated and operating foot controls, fluid stagnates in the feet. Wiggling your toes will help pump the fluid out of your feet and back where it belongs. Pay attention to the position of your toes while driving so that you do not keep your toes curled or extended for any length of time.

To conclude, while commuting by public transportation can't fully replace regular structured workouts, it's a good option if you don't indulge in any exercise whatsoever. So next time you are stuck in a traffic jam, use the time to improve your body. By practicing these simple exercises, you can use your precious time spent going to work. Even if you arrive late, you will look good and feel refreshed when you get there. I hope these ideas provide some inspiration to get the best from your commuting time. Just be sure to stop if you feel unsafe in any way on the road.

# THE OFFICE

If you're one of many who work in an office and find yourself seated at a desk for prolonged periods of time, then you're asking for trouble. The mass office working culture has led to more sedentary lifestyles. Your body is designed for movement, so sitting for long hours at a time doesn't do your body any favors. It's therefore vital that you find ways to move around in order to keep the circulation in your body moving and to keep unwanted fat or weight from creeping up on you. Staying stationary for long periods can also lead to backache, stiffness, and headaches.

If you don't get up and move around every so often, you'll gradually begin to feel uncomfortable, your energy level will decline, and you'll probably feel lethargic and possibly begin to lack concentration resulting in below par productivity.

The great news is this book recognizes these problems. All you need to do is take active steps to solve it. Office exercises are exactly that: an active step. Use office exercises as a way to enjoy your work. Your working life takes up most of your time. If you don't enjoy yours, the chances are you're not enjoying life to its full potential.

At least thirty minutes of moderate exercise five days a week is the recommended amount that you need to maintain a healthy body. However, many of you don't get near enough exercise. Office exercises aren't a total replacement for your regular exercise routine, but they will help to keep you active, burn off the excesses of the day, and, we hope, give you the motivation to partake in a regular exercise program to keep your body trim and healthy.

It's imperative that while seated at your desk you maintain proper posture by keeping your back straight and your shoulders back but comfortably relaxed. If you adopt poor posture when seated, you prevent your lungs from getting adequate oxygen. Also, a good chair designed for desk work or a stability ball is important and will help in improving the way you sit.

The use of a stability ball encourages you to maintain proper spinal alignment in addition to promoting balance and circulation as it allows the blood to flow freely throughout the body. It takes a bit of getting used to sitting on one of these balls, but you'll soon see the benefits if you persevere with it. One good tip is to place a towel over the ball as they can be rather cold! The stability ball is a good tool because it is easy to do a mini-workout while seated on the ball. Most department stores and sporting goods shops stock these balls, but make sure you buy the correct size to suit your height. The information on the outer box will indicate which ball is ideal for you.

Office exercises aren't everyone's cup of tea. You probably do have an open mind, although some of your colleagues may not, so don't be shy when you start doing odd movements!

**CHEST STRETCH:**
Sitting or standing, interlock your fingers behind your back. Making sure your shoulders stay back and down, lift your hands up as far as you can. Relax.

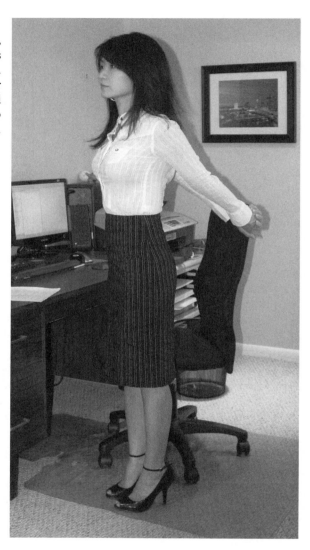

There are plenty of different types of exercises you can do in the office. A lot of it depends on the space you have and what kind of building you're in. Keep them simple and easy to remember. The following are some stretches that you might like to try at your office desk. Slightly increasing your level of activity will aid in increasing your energy level. All it takes is a few minutes a couple times a day to relieve work-related stress, increase your energy level, and ultimately make you healthier. Remember to breathe while you are stretching in order to maximize the benefits of the exercise. You should ideally hold each stretch for a minimum of twenty seconds. Hold for longer if your boss isn't keeping an eye on you!

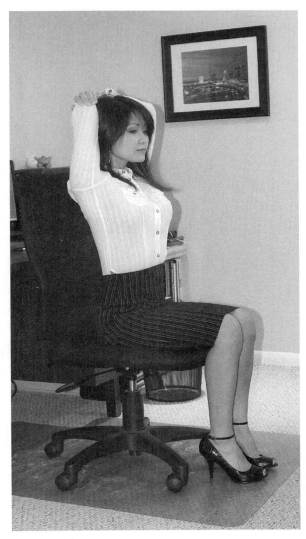

**TRICEPS STRETCH:**
Sitting or standing, bend your right arm back behind your head, so that your palm is between your shoulder blades. Use your left hand to assist the stretch, by pushing your right elbow slightly back. Relax. Repeat with your left arm.

**LOWER BACK STRETCH:**
Sitting in the middle of your chair, both feet flat on the floor. Grip the top of your right knee with both hands, and pull it toward your chest. Repeat with your left knee. Move your head slightly down toward your knee for further stretch.

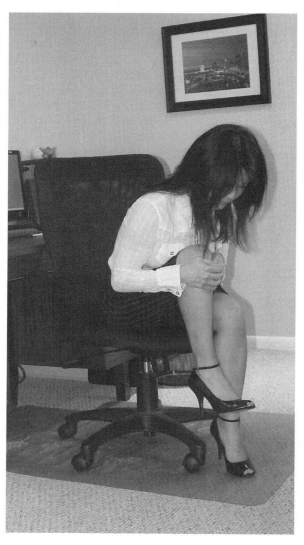

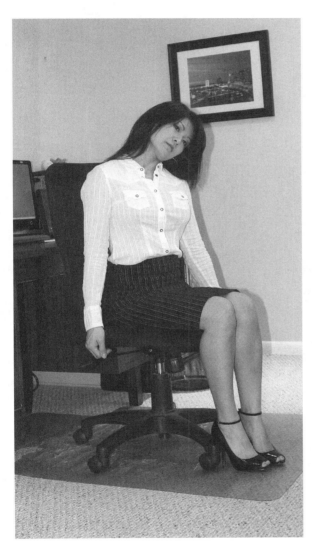

**NECK STRETCHES:**
Slowly tilt your head
toward your shoulder
and hold. Change to
the other side. Ease
into this one slowly and
steadily as the neck is
easy to injure.

**ARM/SHOULDER STRETCH:**
Place your arm across your
chest, hook your other arm
around your elbow to ease
the tension out of your upper
back and rear shoulders.

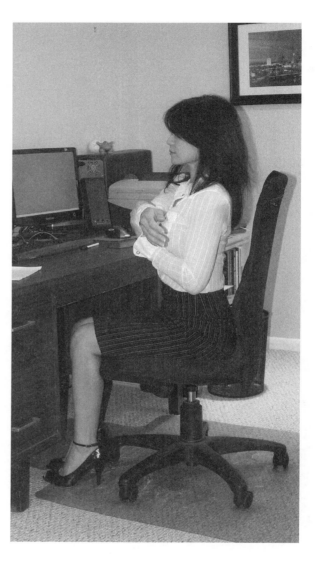

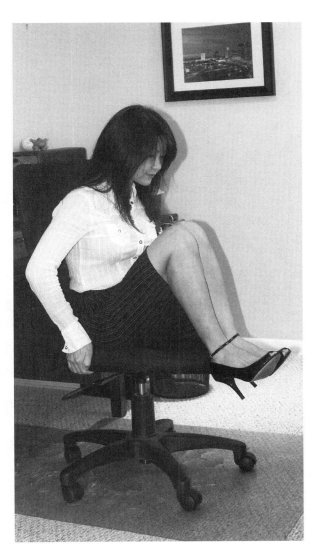

**ABS HOLD:**
Sitting in the middle of your chair, hold the edge of the seat with both hands. Contract your abs while lifting your knees toward your chest (keeping knees together). Relax. Make sure you don't lean back while holding.

**BACK OF LEGS
STRETCH:** Lean forward
at the waist either from
the standing position or
sitting and bring your
chest toward your thighs.
Slowly try to straighten
your legs—stretching your
hamstrings.

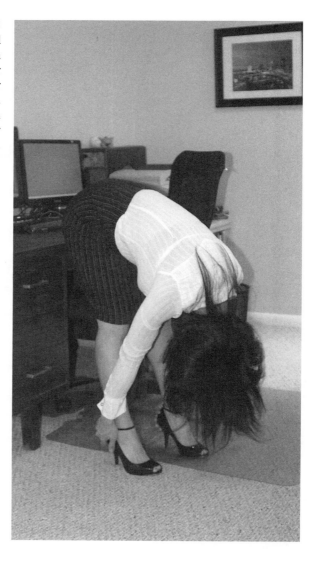

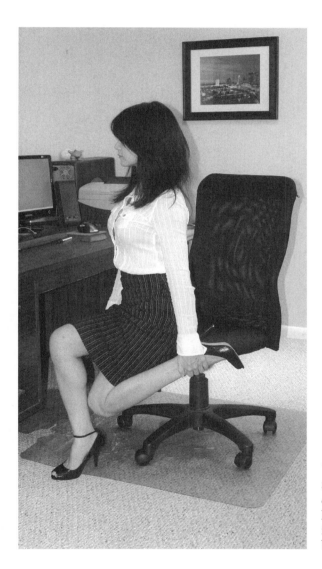

**THIGH STRETCH:**
Sit on the left edge of your chair or stand. Grasp your left ankle and gently pull it up ward toward your buttocks. Switch sides.

**CALVES STRETCH:**
Stand and lean into your desk with your heels on the floor. Bend your knees slightly to stretch your Achilles tendons.

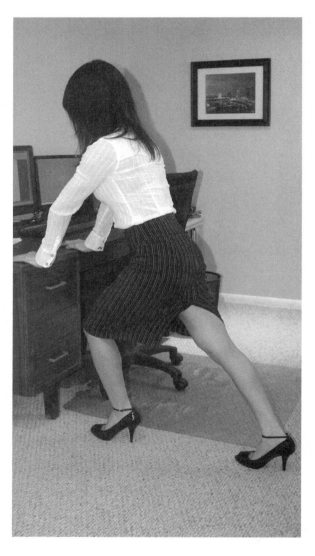

For more dynamic exercises, which involve more movement and that you can do around common office areas (e.g., empty conference room, photocopy room, or stairwell), check out the exercises below. They should be performed in a controlled and un-rushed manner. Make sure you warm up prior to starting these with a few mobility exercises or a gentle stair walk first. Add a few more repetitions if you feel comfortable.

## MESSAGE IN PERSON:
At work, try to communicate with your colleagues face-to-face as much as possible. Instead of using the phone or e-mail to send a message, simply walk to your coworker's desk or office. Not only will you earn valuable steps throughout the day, but you might start a trend in your workplace.

## STAIR WALKING:
Walk up and down a few flights of stairs several times. You can increase the intensity by taking two stair steps at a time. This will "fire up" your thighs and buttock muscles to make them work harder.

## SIDE-STEPPING STAIR WALKING:
Walk up and down the stairs as before, but this time start walking sideways up first! Try walking a whole flight of stairs with your right side leading, then swap over to the other side for the next flight of stairs. When you reach the top, do the same again on the descent.

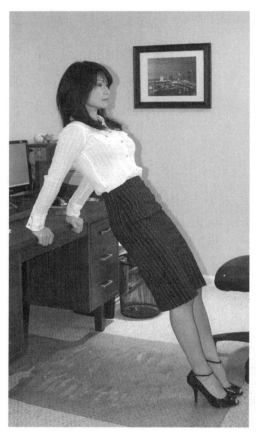

## BENCH DIPS:

Using your chair or a sturdy table, place your hands on the edge and bend your arms to slowly lower yourself until your arms are at a right angle. Raise yourself by extending your arms. Aim to achieve ten to fifteen repetitions.

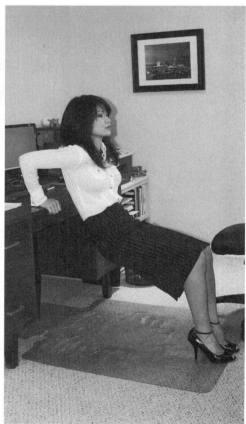

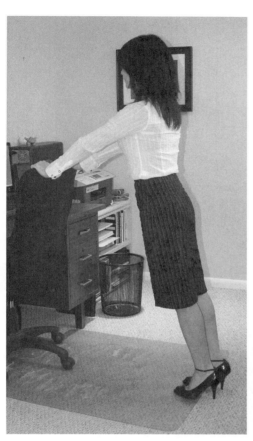

### ASSISTED PUSH-UP:

In the office, you can do push-ups anywhere there's a solid object—against the wall, desk, or door frame. For example, lean up against your desk and push yourself away from the desk while in a leaning position. Ensure that your chest touches the desk for maximum effect. Aim to achieve ten to fifteen repetitions.

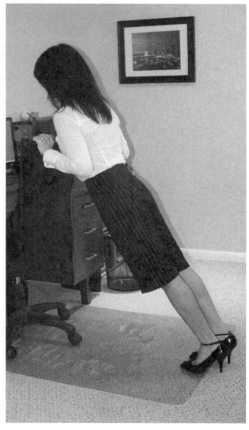

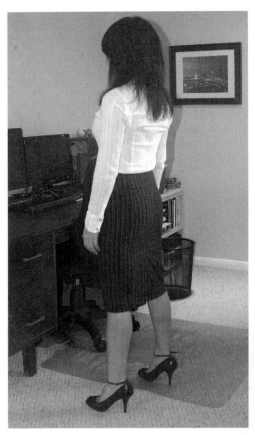

## LEG SQUATS:

In a standing position with your feet shoulder-width apart, bend your knees in position, so your bottom goes back and down. Extend your legs to return to the start position. Aim to achieve ten to fifteen repetitions.

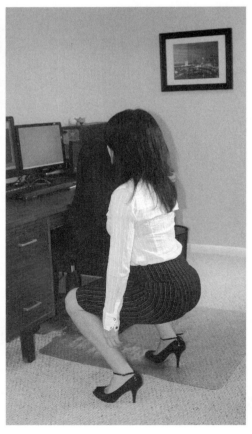

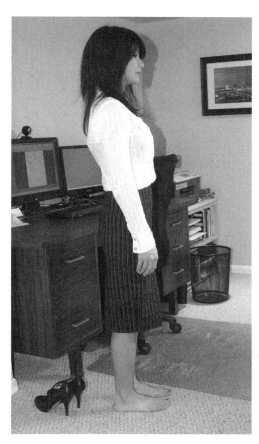

## CALF RAISES:

 Stand up and place your hands on your hips for balance. Now raise all body weight onto the balls of your feet. Slowly lower until your feet are flat on the floor again. Aim to achieve ten to fifteen repetitions.

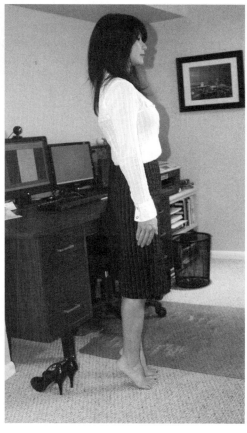

## EXERCISING IN YOUR OFFICE IS ABOUT MAKING LIFE EASIER FOR YOURSELF.

Whether you're having a good or bad day in the office, any sort of exercise will make you feel better. A few minutes of office exercise will refresh concentration and relieve muscles. So break up your workday to include some or all of these simple, yet effective exercises. It all leads to a more productive and healthier you.

While I was writing this book, I sat on my stability ball and set an alarm clock to remind me to get moving every thirty minutes!

***Please Note: Consider your company's health and safety regulations when doing any of these office exercises.***

Though most of the activities and movements covered in this chapter are designed for different locations or times of day, they all share one thing in common: these are all simple lifestyle changes that can exist as healthy parts of a larger lifestyle change. Most importantly, consider that these tips represent only a few ways to integrate exercise into your daily life. Based on your daily routine and new healthy lifestyle, you may find that the opportunities to sneak exercise into your life are limitless!

# CHAPTER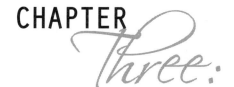

## FIT YOUR BUDGET

CHAPTER THREE:
# FIT YOUR *budget*

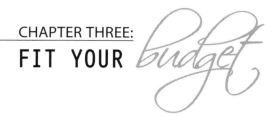

U ndecided about whether to exercise at home or continue with your
gym membership? Both locations are versatile and offer unlimited
workout options, but if you like to workout far from the madding crowds
in a more private environment, then ditching your fitness club membership
in favor of exercising at home will result in substantial savings over time.
Not everyone can afford a costly gym membership. Even if a membership is
within your budget, often you'll find yourself waiting in line to get to use the
equipment, especially on crowded days. This can really set a workout routine
out of kilter.

## TO BUY OR NOT TO BUY — THAT IS THE QUESTION!

There are many other benefits to be had from the *Celebrity Body on a Budget*
home workouts. It doesn't have to be hell to be healthy, and it needn't cost a
fortune either. While some people love the buzz of going to the gym, others
prefer to exercise in private. Fitness clubs provide the advantage of working
out with other like-minded individuals. And if you are the type of person who
needs inspiration from others, the fitness club provides that environment.
Of course, if you're the socially inclined type, it's also a great place to meet
others. If exercise for you is not a social activity and you want to burn as many
calories and tone as many muscles in as little time as possible, exercising using
the home exercise equipment guide can be just as practical.

There's a tremendous range of home fitness equipment available.
Choose your equipment with care, and you'll have all the ingredients to
construct a balanced, all-over body training program, all in your own lounge,
spare room, or garage.

Depending on how far away your gym is you could be spending a substantial
amount of time every week driving back and forth to work out. By purchasing
and installing home fitness equipment, you can continue to get a solid
workout in the privacy of your own home without having to travel to your
fitness center and paying ongoing membership fees. Think of all the time and
money you will save by eliminating the drive to the gym every day and paying
your monthly dues. The cost of a good quality exercise machine is estimated
to be the equivalent of six to ten months of an average gym membership
subscription.

So, if you've put off purchasing home fitness equipment because of price or space, now is the best time to grab a bargain on a piece of equipment that will last for years. Here's your chance to look over the list of the best home fitness equipment and see how affordable it is to get started on building a stronger, healthier you.

Home fitness machines are typically accompanied by exercise guides. Some manufacturers go one step further by throwing in an exercise DVD or video that teaches you how to use your piece of equipment. By following these instructions, you don't need a personal trainer to instruct you like in a fitness center.

## AT YOUR LEISURE

By opting for home fitness equipment, you'll also be buying convenience. You will appreciate the privacy and convenience of owning quality exercise equipment that you can use any time you feel like working out. You'll save time and won't have to stand in line to use the machines at the fitness club. You can utilize your time much better with home training devices because you can do your workout routines while your food is cooking, or even when having conversations with your family or friends whether it be face-to-face or on the telephone. If you place your exercise equipment near your TV, you can even do your complete exercise routine while watching your favorite shows or catching up on the daily news.

If you decide to follow this path, you'll first need to consider which kind of exercise equipment you'll need. Your workout plan determines exactly which kind of training you are going to do and the equipment that is necessary for this kind of workout.

It's no new discovery that the best way to attain the leanest, most defined muscles is through a combination of aerobic exercise and resistance training, so let's take a look at what you need to perform such training.

For aerobic exercise, which is the best way to lose fat and build cardiovascular endurance, all you need is twenty minutes of exercise per day with no equipment at all. Of course, if you want to vary your aerobic training, you can buy an exercise bike, rower, treadmill, ski machine, elliptical machine, etc., which will substitute for any equipment you've used at your gym.

Incorporating resistance exercises into your exercise program builds muscle and tone. Resistance training requires a little more equipment, however, and the most important here are various weights. You can also use home fitness machines for resistance training. There are some combination machines on the market that can take care of all your weight and/or resistance training needs, for all your muscles in your entire body. These are known as multigyms, and the prices can be reasonable. Naturally, there are some quality differences, and it normally pays to buy quality training equipment, especially if you are going to train for the long term. As in most cases, you must weigh what a piece of equipment costs by how many years you'll be able to use it.

Sourcing the best home fitness equipment and deciding which one is right for you can sometimes seem a daunting task. You want to get value for money as well as find the best deal in a quality system that will endure your workouts. There's never been a more exciting time to purchase a home gym. Today's equipment are better designed and more compact, more versatile, made with better quality materials, and, best of all, even with all the advancements in design, they have never been more affordable than now!

In addition to circuit machines and other multistation home gyms, you can explore what is available in abdominal exercise machines and cardio fitness equipment. Since everyone's needs are different, this section of the book will tell how you can install a custom home gym. If you are on a budget (and who isn't?), this book offers a guide to buying compact, used, and discount home gyms.

## CONSIDER THIS

The increasingly popular fitness market is full of different types of home fitness equipment. When you decide to buy your own home gym equipment, you will likely struggle to determine what is the best way to go about doing it. Should you buy new home fitness equipment or used equipment? Should you start with only one piece of equipment or purchase a few? What brand of equipment is the most reliable? If you've settled on buying something that you believe is ideal for you, wait until you know a little more because the last thing you want to do is return it because it isn't really what you wanted. Fitness equipment should never be bought on a whim. If you are unsure about your plans, always carefully consider your motives for buying it first.

## HASTE MAKES WASTE

It is easy to be tempted when you see home fitness equipment advertised on television, but these infomercials don't have time to tell the whole truth. Ask yourself a few questions before you grab your credit card and the phone and buy that equipment; it could save you hassle and money. No one wants to waste money, and some home fitness equipment can be expensive. You'll need to assess what it is you want to get out of the equipment. Ideally, you will have tried the equipment out first at a sports equipment store or an equivalent machine at your gym.

If you decide that working out at home makes the most sense, the first consideration will be the location. You may choose the basement. But if it is dark and damp, this isn't an inspiring environment. Another consideration is an extra bedroom or part of a family room or playroom. You want an inviting location that is well ventilated and provides sufficient light. For those who like to keep up with the latest news or the music channels, a room with a television would be idyllic. If lack of space is a consideration, there is fitness equipment such as folding treadmills or compact home gyms that minimize required space.

Think about whether your intended exercise equipment is safe for you to use, particularly if you have existing medical conditions. Check with your doctor to assess if it is suitable for you to use a piece of equipment, before you buy it. If the equipment is unfamiliar to you, make sure you test it first because you do not want to have a piece of apparatus you find uncomfortable to use.

You may be lucky enough to locate a fitness equipment retailer willing to offer a try-before-you-buy deal for a few weeks, which gives you the opportunity to "test drive" a range of equipment. Compared to the money you will spend if you buy an unsuitable item of home fitness equipment and end up hating it, this can sometimes be the best option. Companies that offer exercise equipment for hire are growing in popularity. They'll charge you a monthly fee with a minimum rental term and deliver and set up your chosen equipment. You can decide to keep the item or exchange it for another machine at the end of your agreed term. The monthly rental costs can often be tantamount to a gym membership, so this option may not be the most cost efficient, although you'll save on time and travel.

Don't be led to believe that if you spend a great deal of money on your new fitness apparatus, it will be incentive enough to use it. The cost should never be the reason it will be used.

Once you have set yourself a budget, find the best equipment you can—either new or used—for the amount you have available. Think quality. And remember, quality doesn't have to break the bank. While it's easy to spend hundreds and even thousands of dollars on home exercise equipment, a far more modest outlay can give equal, and frequently, greater training benefits. An investment of $50 to $90 will provide you with everything you need to get started and enjoy comprehensive, total body training sessions covering cardio, flexibility, resistance training for toning, and coordination. Some basic dumbbells, an exercise mat, a stability ball, and a jump rope provide a cheap, simple "home gym," on which you can always expand at a later date.

## IN WITH THE OLD OR OUT WITH THE NEW?

Not all home fitness equipment has to be expensive. You can get some great discount home fitness equipment as well. If price is an issue when opting for your own home fitness gym, take a look around for some discount equipment to get you started. There's no written rule that brand new home fitness equipment is a must to get a great workout. You can realize substantial savings if you're prepared to source used equipment. Trawling through the classified advertisements in your local newspaper or on the Web (eBay, Craig's List) can be a bargain hunter's delight. More often than not, secondhand exercise equipment can be obtained for a fraction of their original cost. Sometimes the owner in need of de-cluttering his home is more than happy to recycle by giving away his unwanted fitness equipment—for free.

You may even strike it lucky and discover that you can buy a used piece of equipment that's never seen daylight and still in its original packaging. These are usually unwanted gifts, and some may have only been used a few times and feel like new. Similarly, if you've found that your recently acquired secondhand equipment isn't up to par or doesn't match your needs, then you can always sell it for more or less than what you paid for it without suffering a substantial loss on your investment.

Then again, not all used equipment is suitable for resale. Be careful not to be coaxed into buying something that was owned by an enthusiastic exerciser who spent the last six months adding several thousand miles on that bit of equipment. It's a simple case of buyer beware.

As most pieces of home fitness equipment are quite sizable and weigh a significant amount, many find that buying new home fitness equipment makes the most sense because they can take advantage of the retailer's delivery options. Setting up and installing some of the more sophisticated machines requires a fair degree of mechanical skills. Therefore, depending on where the equipment is purchased from, delivery may include setup and installation of your new equipment, which could prove to be a valuable service.

Another reason to purchase new home fitness equipment is that the life span of new equipment may be much longer than that of used equipment. Consider how often you want to replace your equipment. By investing more money up front, you can save yourself the trouble of sourcing, transporting, and installing used equipment every few years.

If you prefer to have new home fitness equipment with a guarantee, then start your search with ex-demonstration stock used in stores or the previous generation models that may be sold for less as the newer model is about to arrive. This is probably the most sensible and cost-effective approach to acquiring the equipment you really want at a price that you can afford.

On the hygiene front, working out can be a sweaty ordeal and would you want to inherit another person's sweat? This reason alone deters a large number of people from going to a gym in the first place or from acquiring used equipment.

Finally, whether you rent or buy new, discounted, or used equipment, you may still find yourself investing quite a bit of money in your home gym, but you will ultimately be investing in yourself. By purchasing the best home fitness equipment, you can ensure that it will be durable enough to withstand your vigorous workouts. Be cautious about wasting money on low-quality fitness equipment that breaks after a few uses—look for quality in both new and used equipment.

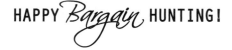

HAPPY *Bargain* HUNTING!

## THE CELEBRITY BODY ON A BUDGET
## DIRECTORY OF HOME EXERCISE EQUIPMENT

Exercising at home can be rewarding, and there is a vast range of home exercise equipment available, from fitness club standard equipment to much more basic, yet functional gear. In general, the more features home gym equipment has, the more parts of your body it exercises. This book has taken the sweat out of choosing home exercise equipment. We give you the low-down on functional products that'll improve your fitness but won't significantly dent your bank account. Now let's take a closer analysis of the different type of machines available in today's marketplace.

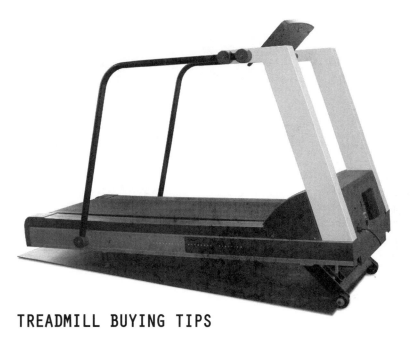

## TREADMILL BUYING TIPS

Treadmills (a.k.a. running machines) remain the most popular home fitness equipment. All you need to know to use a treadmill is how to walk or run—the treadmill takes care of the rest. When you love the workout you get from a run or brisk walk but just can't get outside, treadmills are the machines for you. They will allow you to burn calories, build muscle, lose weight, and strengthen your heart and lungs.

### FEATURES TO LOOK FOR IN TREADMILLS
Many treadmills allow you set the speed and incline for your walk or run, but if you'd rather not deal with a lot of settings, you can select a manual treadmill. If you want to put away your treadmill after your workout, choose a folding treadmill so you can slide it under the bed or into a closet.

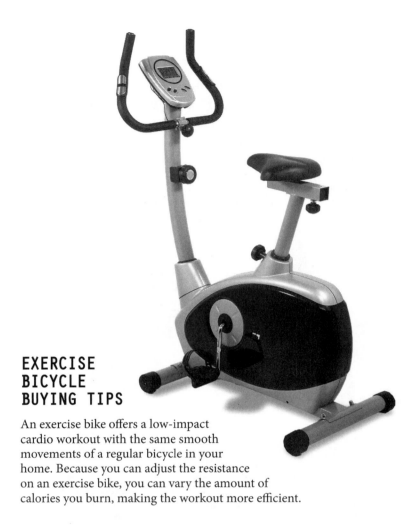

## EXERCISE BICYCLE BUYING TIPS

An exercise bike offers a low-impact cardio workout with the same smooth movements of a regular bicycle in your home. Because you can adjust the resistance on an exercise bike, you can vary the amount of calories you burn, making the workout more efficient.

### FEATURES TO LOOK FOR IN EXERCISE BIKES

All exercise bicycles should allow you to adjust the seat to ensure a proper fit. You will have various ways to adjust the tension on an exercise bike. Some require you to stop and get off the stationary bike, while others can be adjusted during your workout. There are three different kinds of exercise bicycles.

1. An upright exercise bike lets you sit in the same upright position as a regular bicycle.

2. A recumbent bike lets you sit back with the pedals more in front of you instead of underneath you. This creates a comfortable workout if you suffer with back pain.

3. A dual-action stationary bike has handles you can move while you pedal providing you with an upper and lower body workout simultaneously.

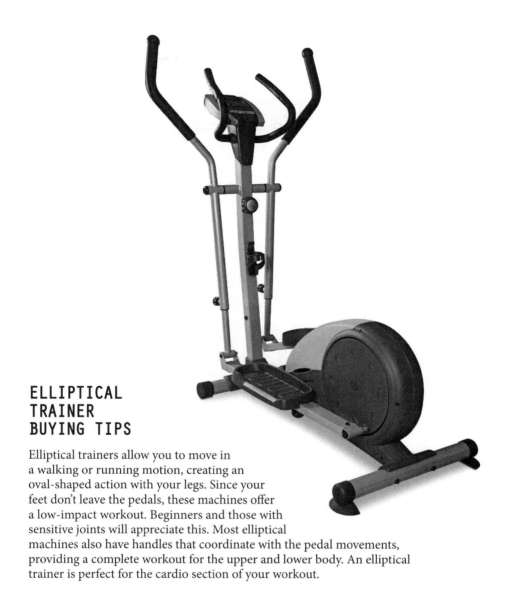

## ELLIPTICAL TRAINER BUYING TIPS

Elliptical trainers allow you to move in a walking or running motion, creating an oval-shaped action with your legs. Since your feet don't leave the pedals, these machines offer a low-impact workout. Beginners and those with sensitive joints will appreciate this. Most elliptical machines also have handles that coordinate with the pedal movements, providing a complete workout for the upper and lower body. An elliptical trainer is perfect for the cardio section of your workout.

### FEATURES TO LOOK FOR IN AN ELLIPTICAL TRAINER

Most elliptical trainers require electricity or batteries to power the monitor, but the movement is mainly driven with your feet and partially with your arms. If you would like to use your elliptical in forward or reverse motions, find one that will do both. Although most elliptical trainers include moving handles, you can find some with stationary handles as well. Many handles also include heart rate monitors. Make sure the size of the elliptical can accommodate your stride length. More expensive models have adjustable stride lengths, which are also designed to increase your calorie burn.

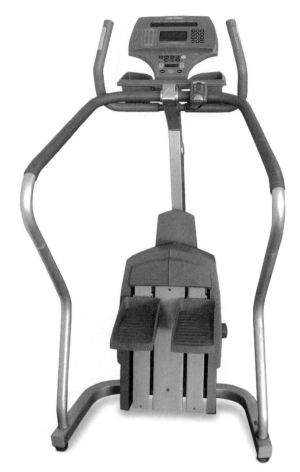

## STEPPING MACHINE BUYING TIPS

A stepping machine (or stepper as it is sometimes called) is another piece of equipment that offers intense, high calorie-burning, low-impact exercise and has remained one of the most popular fitness products available. Not only is a stepping machine easy to set up, take down, and store, but it is simplicity itself. Step training can be a tough, athletic challenge, but it offers positive results on buttocks and thigh strength. A high-intensity workout can be achieved and maintained more quickly by step training than traditional aerobic exercise and, as a result, provides the necessary cardiovascular workload needed to attain desired training effects.

### FEATURES TO LOOK FOR IN A STEPPING MACHINE

Step training is also a relatively simple form of exercise with arm and step patterns adding creativity and style to the workout. The stepper replaces the traditional step bench with modern functions such as a heart rate monitor, a selection of different workout programs, variable resistance, and digital displays. If you don't have a great deal of room, there are even mini-step machines.

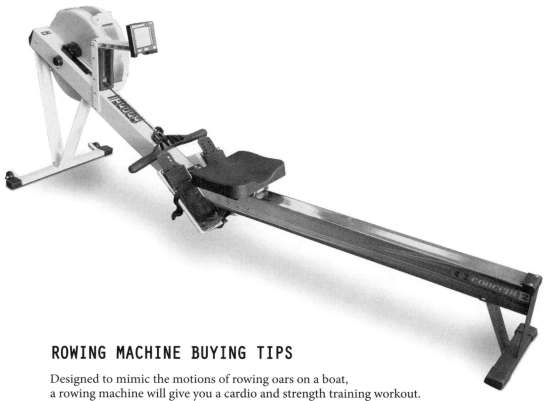

## ROWING MACHINE BUYING TIPS

Designed to mimic the motions of rowing oars on a boat,
a rowing machine will give you a cardio and strength training workout.
This is a full body workout that will increase muscle tone in your back, arms,
legs, and core. Because of the exertion required, rowing machines aren't as
popular as some other home exercise equipment, and a rowing machine may
be unsuitable if you suffer with bad knees or back problems. However, the
workout intensity of a row machine is appreciated by people who are serious
about getting
into shape.

### FEATURES TO LOOK FOR IN A ROWING MACHINE

The main difference you'll find between different rowing machines is the
resistance that simulates the rowing action. Some row machines use a
combination of these methods, and most offer adjustable resistance:

**Hydraulic piston:**  Pistons are the least expensive method, but new models
allow for a smooth, natural movement.

**Air:** Air pressure creates resistance. This type of rowing machine is the most
common. It is durable but can be more expensive.

**Magnetic:** The quietest of all the rowing machines, the magnetic row machine
does not use a flywheel. It is also smooth.

**Water:** A flywheel in water gives a realistic rowing experience. This can be
somewhat noisy, but many people find the water sound to be soothing.

## JUMP ROPE

Jump ropes or skipping ropes are inexpensive, small, and portable. They offer a scalable workout that can be easy or extremely challenging, depending upon your fitness level and goals. Jumping rope for just a few minutes a day is as good for your heart as a thirty-minute jog. It can be a nice break to a regular exercise routine.

### FEATURES TO LOOK FOR IN A JUMP ROPE

They're available in varying lengths and materials from special plastic (speed ropes) to real cotton rope and real leather.

Some even come with a clever digital "Skip" counter that records the number of revolutions and/or calories burned.

Optional weighted handles for a more efficient workout are also available on some of the expensive ropes.

## STRENGTH TRAINING AND SPECIFIC TRAINING MACHINES

The strength training portion of your workout allows you to focus on creating tone and muscle strength. When your muscles are in shape, your lean muscle will burn calories even while you rest, you'll be able to perform better, you'll reduce pain and risk of injury, and you will reduce your risk of developing many diseases, including heart disease, diabetes, and osteoporosis.

## WEIGHTS AND WEIGHT MACHINES

No home gym is complete without a few weights. Weight training helps you work on your strength, and there are weights to work each of your muscle groups. You can add hand weights or leg weights to your cardio workout to increase the resistance or use the weights separately. While dumbbell sets are versatile, a weight machine gives you even more options for weight training.

### FEATURES TO LOOK FOR IN WEIGHT TRAINING MACHINES

· An adjustable bench to accommodate all who will use the weight machine.

· A variety of exercises so you can work each muscle group.

· Enough weight to give you the workout you want.

You can choose between weight training machines with stacked weights or strong and durable rubber bands to create resistance.

You can also decide if you want a weight machine with a few stations so multiple people can use it at once.

Weight machines that can fold up for easy storage are also available.

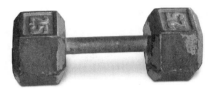

## DUMBBELLS AND BARBELLS

These come in many shapes, sizes, and weights. You can buy adjustable dumbbells and barbells that are more compact and easier to store; these tend to be a little more expensive though. There are also many small sets of dumbbells available in various weight ranges; alternatively, they can be bought individually.

Resistance bands are without a doubt the most versatile, budget-friendly piece of home fitness equipment. They are also the easiest to store away when not in use. When buying resistance bands, it's recommended that you buy more than one strength. Most manufacturers offer three or four different strengths ranging from light to heavy.

## CHIN-UP/PULL-UP BAR

Pull-ups and chin-ups encourage you to lift your own body weight. They are excellent for a strength building workout especially for your upper back structure. Unfortunately, pull-ups and chin-ups are hard. Very hard. If you're a beginner, chances are you may not be able to do even one pull-up or chin-up. When used regularly, however, you'll soon get stronger at doing them, so you'll eventually be able to complete sets.

You also can use your doorway chin-up bar for abdominal exercises. Just hang by your hands and raise your knees to waist level to mimic knee raises. It's tough but effective. This is another example of the versatility of chin-up bars.

Chin-up bars are designed to be fitted in between your doorframe and are secured into place by end brackets. It's easy to install the bar, but make sure it is secure before using it.

## ABDOMINAL MACHINES

An ab machine lets you focus on the muscles in the center of your stomach and on the sides. Although the movements are similar to sit-ups or crunches, an ab machine adds resistance to increase the effectiveness of each move. These machines should be adjustable to your body size to avoid injuries. One thing to consider with an ab machine is: it will not decrease the fat on your stomach, but it will help tone muscles. You need to combine the use of your ab machine with a cardio workout to burn the fat.

## PILATES EXERCISE EQUIPMENT

Pilates exercise equipment helps you perform a Pilates workout with the precision that Pilates creator Joseph Pilates intended. If you need to add flexibility training to your workout, the stretching you'll do with Pilates exercise equipment will be a great addition to your home gym. You also can add strength training and core training with Pilates exercise equipment.

## VIBRATION EQUIPMENT

Currently, the trendiest piece of fitness equipment is vibration equipment. Essentially, it is a vibrating plate that activates muscle contractions much quicker than traditional training methods. The result is that you work against a far greater influence or "load" of gravity in every movement you perform.

## FITNESS DVDS

For a low investment, you can get your favorite celebrity or your very own personal trainer in your living room. The right DVD should provide a safe, balanced, and interesting workout. Choose a fitness DVD that you won't get bored with or outgrow too quickly. Before you buy a DVD, sample it for free by checking out the selections at your local library. There are also plenty of fitness DVDs on the secondhand market (E-bay springs to mind).

This is a just a short list of potential home fitness equipment. It can be supplemented with the current generation of computer-aided exercise devices and countless other exercise devices and products.

# CHAPTER
*Four:*

## ANALYZE THIS
### (PERSONAL FITNESS EVALUATION)      67

# CHAPTER FOUR:

# ANALYZE *this*

## (PERSONAL FITNESS EVALUATION)

To get anywhere, you need to know where you're starting from, and this very much applies to your body and what shape it's in. By completing your own fitness evaluation at home, you can quickly and easily establish your overall physical condition. At first, this can be daunting for some people because the results often confirm what they already suspect—that they are carrying more weight than necessary, that they are out of condition, and worse still, that they can be at risk of ill health. Assessing your own fitness is not akin to an exam where you pass or fail. It should be viewed as providing a "benchmark" from which to start.

Before you begin the self fitness test, you should invest a few minutes in completing the questionnaire in this chapter. Once you've completed this, you're then ready to take the fitness test. This is comprised of some simple tests, and not only will it help you to evaluate your current fitness level, but it will help you to decide what program of exercise is most suited to you. These tests are not too difficult or time consuming. Try to enjoy the challenge and the results will reveal to you a lot about your overall physical condition.

As you take up a regular exercise program and begin realizing the benefits of using this book, you will want to periodically test your progress. Although you will feel better as a result of a lifestyle change, these changes are sometimes hard to recognize because they occur gradually. That's why I recommend that you retest yourself every two to three months. Not only will it reveal your progress, but it will give you confidence that will you are improving your overall condition. As your results and scores improve, you'll enjoy a greater sense of accomplishment and satisfaction. I have deliberately provided space on some of the pages for you to record your values for each test.

# PRE-EXERCISE QUESTIONNAIRE

Start off by reading all of the questions first. Be honest with yourself and think each one through carefully before answering them. Check the most appropriate statement that you think best describes you. The numbers in brackets indicate your sub-scores for each question that you answer. Let's start!

## Age: Which age category do you fall into?

___ Below the age of 20—(3)

___ Ages 21 to 30—(2)

___ Ages 31 to 40—(1)

___ Age 41 and up—0)

## Cardiovascular Health: This relates to the health of your heart and respiratory system.

___ I do not have any history of heart or lung disease within myself or immediate family—(3)

___ I have had successful treatment in the past, and the doctor has given me the all clear—(2)

___ I have an existing problem, but am no longer receiving treatment—(1)

___ I'm currently under medical supervision—(0)

## Injuries: These questions relate to the condition of your muscles and joints.

___ I'm current injury free—(3)

___ I have recovered from an old past injury, with no recurrence—(2)

___ I am recovering from a recent injury—(1)

___ I presently am suffering from a painful injury—(0)

## Illness: Choose the statement that closely describes your overall health.

___ I am in good general health, with no signs of illness—(3)

___ I am suffering mildly from ill health, but recovering—(2)

___ I am particularly limited by illness—(1)

___ I am unable to do much without feeling the effect of my illness—(0)

**Weight: You will need to weigh yourself first using accurate scales. Then using a weight chart, determine your ideal weight.**

___ I am within 2 pounds of my correct weight—(3)

___ I am within 9 pounds of my correct weight—(2)

___ I am 10 to 19 pounds above or below my correct weight—(1)

___ I am 20 pounds or more above or below my correct weight—(0)

**Lifestyle: These questions address aspects of your normal daily life.**

___ I currently do not smoke and never have—(3)

___ I used to smoke but have now quit—(2)

___ I am a social, occasional smoker—(1)

___ I smoke regularly and have done so for more than one year—(0)

**Food: Daily food intake consisting of three balanced meals that includes fresh produce, lean meat, poultry, fish, complex carbohydrates, and water.**

___ I eat 3 regular, healthy balanced meals each day that includes all of the above—(3)

___ I skip the odd meal here and there with only a few pieces of fresh produce and limited water intake—(2)

___ I eat lunch and evening meals only and do not always make sensible choices—(1)

___ I am erratic, eating mainly ready-made meals with no fresh produce, washed down with beer—(0)

**Exercise: To reap the rewards of exercise, you should be aiming to be physically active on almost a daily basis.**

___ I am presently exercising fairly briskly 3 or more times a week—(3)

___ I am physically active with walking the dog and doing house chores on most days—(2)

___ Occasionally, I participate in the odd game of sport or go for a walk—(1)

___ I have a totally sedentary lifestyle with no exercise whatsoever—(0)

# THE PERSONAL FITNESS & MONITORING TEST

If you experience any discomfort, dizziness, or nausea throughout the physical working aspects of this fitness test, then discontinue and consult your doctor.

## HEIGHT TO WEIGHT CHARTS

**Weight without Clothes; Height without Shoes**

**Ideal Height/Weight Chart**

## WEIGHT TABLES FOR MEN IN POUNDS

| Height | Small frame | Medium frame | Large frame |
|--------|-------------|--------------|-------------|
| 5'2" | 128-134 | 131-141 | 138-150 |
| 5'3" | 130-136 | 133-143 | 140-153 |
| 5'4" | 132-138 | 135-145 | 142-156 |
| 5'5" | 134-140 | 137-148 | 144-160 |
| 5'6" | 136-142 | 139-151 | 146-164 |
| 5'7" | 138-145 | 142-154 | 149-168 |
| 5'8" | 140-148 | 145-157 | 152-172 |
| 5'9" | 142-151 | 148-160 | 155-176 |
| 5'10" | 144-154 | 151-163 | 158-180 |
| 5'11" | 146-157 | 154-166 | 161-184 |
| 6'0" | 149-160 | 157-170 | 164-188 |
| 6'1" | 152-164 | 160-174 | 168-192 |
| 6'2" | 155-168 | 164-178 | 172-197 |
| 6'3" | 158-172 | 167-182 | 176-202 |
| 6'4" | 162-176 | 171-187 | 181-207 |

## WEIGHT TABLES FOR WOMEN IN POUNDS

| Height | Small frame | Medium frame | Large frame |
|--------|-------------|--------------|-------------|
| 4'10" | 102-111 | 109-121 | 118-131 |
| 4'11" | 103-113 | 111-123 | 120-134 |
| 5'0" | 104-115 | 113-126 | 122-137 |
| 5'1" | 106-118 | 115-129 | 125-140 |
| 5'2" | 108-121 | 118-132 | 128-143 |
| 5'3" | 111-124 | 121-135 | 131-147 |
| 5'4" | 114-127 | 124-138 | 134-151 |
| 5'5" | 117-130 | 127-141 | 137-155 |
| 5'6" | 120-133 | 130-144 | 140-159 |
| 5'7" | 123-136 | 133-147 | 143-163 |
| 5'8" | 126-139 | 136-150 | 146-167 |
| 5'9" | 129-142 | 139-153 | 149-170 |
| 5'10" | 132-145 | 142-156 | 152-173 |
| 5'11" | 135-148 | 145-159 | 155-176 |
| 6'0" | 138-151 | 148-162 | 158-179 |

**Make a note of your body weight measurements here:**

Date/Weight: _____

Date/Weight: _____

Date/Weight: _____

## BODY DIMENSIONS

Review your body dimensions periodically and record them on the chart.

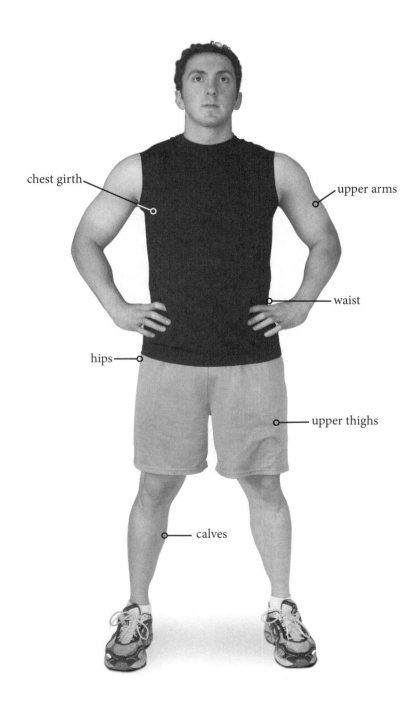

chest girth

upper arms

waist

hips

upper thighs

calves

## BODY MASS INDEX TEST (BMI)

Procedure: This is a more accurate method of determining the correct weight for your height. It is defined as your body weight in kilograms divided by your height in meters squared. The recommended BMI for men is set between 21-26, while in women it is 18-23. See the chart below as a quick reference to work out your own BMI. To the right of the chart, you can note the categories that will apply to your finding.

## BMI FORMULA:

$$\text{BMI} = \left( \frac{\text{(Weight in Pounds)}}{\text{(Height in Inches)} \times \text{(Height in Inches)}} \right) \times 703$$

*For example, for a man of 5 feet 10 inches tall (70 inches) and weighing 180 pounds, the calculation would be:*

$$\text{BMI} = \left( \frac{180 \text{ (Weight in Pounds)}}{4900 \text{ (70 Inches)} \times \text{(70 Inches)}} \right) \times 703 = 25.82$$

## BODY MASS INDEX CHART

| Body Mass Index (BMI) | | | | | | |
|---|---|---|---|---|---|---|
| Weight (pounds) | Height (feet, inches) | | | | | |
| | 5'0" | 5'3" | 5'6" | 5'9" | 6'0" | 6'3" |
| 140 | 27 | 25 | 23 | 21 | 19 | 18 |
| 150 | 29 | 27 | 24 | 22 | 20 | 19 |
| 160 | 31 | 28 | 26 | 24 | 22 | 20 |
| 170 | 33 | 30 | 27 | 25 | 23 | 21 |
| 180 | 35 | 32 | 29 | 27 | 25 | 23 |
| 190 | 37 | 34 | 31 | 28 | 26 | 24 |
| 200 | 39 | 35 | 32 | 30 | 27 | 25 |
| 210 | 41 | 37 | 34 | 31 | 28 | 26 |
| 220 | 43 | 39 | 36 | 33 | 30 | 27 |
| 230 | 45 | 41 | 37 | 34 | 31 | 29 |
| 240 | 47 | 43 | 39 | 35 | 33 | 30 |
| 250 | 49 | 44 | 40 | 37 | 34 | 31 |

## BMI RATING AND SCORES ARE AS FOLLOWS:

### Men

| | |
|---|---|
| 21-26: | Normal—(3) |
| 27-30: | Below normal—(2) |
| 31-35: | Poor—(1) |
| 36-40: | Very poor—(0) |

### Women

| | |
|---|---|
| 18-23: | Normal—(3) |
| 24-27: | Below normal—(2) |
| 28-32: | Poor—(1) |
| 33-37: | Very poor—(0) |

**Record your BMI readings here:**

Date/Index:_____

Date/Index:_____

Date/Index:_____

## CHECKING YOUR FAT LEVELS

____ I have a flat stomach coupled with no love handles—(3)

____ I can pinch more than 1 inch, but less than 2 inches on any part of waist line—(2)

____ I can grab more than a handful of soft flesh from my "love handles"—(1)

____ From a standing position, I can't see my toes without bending forward—(0)

# TESTING YOUR CARDIOVASCULAR FITNESS

Resting Heart Rate (BPM=beats per minute)

## HOW TO MEASURE YOUR HEART RATE

Procedure: Before you begin this test, ensure that you have become proficient at checking your pulse rate manually (see the section on aerobic exercise in chapter 1). Sit down in a comfortable armchair. Avoid any excitable or stressful distractions whether environmental or emotional. Wait a few minutes and then check your resting heart rate. You may wish to try it a few times over a ten-minute period. If you receive varying readings, then take an average of your findings.

## RATINGS AND SCORE/VALUES:

60 BPM or below = Excellent (score 4)
61-70 BPM    = Good (3)
71-75 BPM    = Average (2)
76-80 BPM    = Below average (1)
81-90 BPM    = Poor (0)

**Note your resting heart rate (RHR) readings here:**

Date/RHR:_____

Date/RHR:_____

Date/RHR:_____

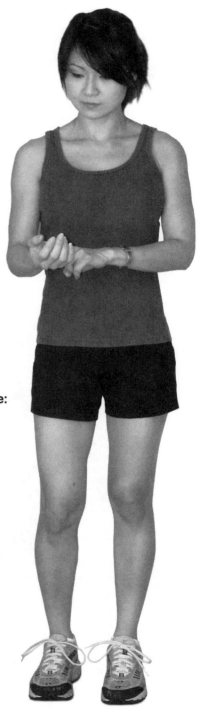

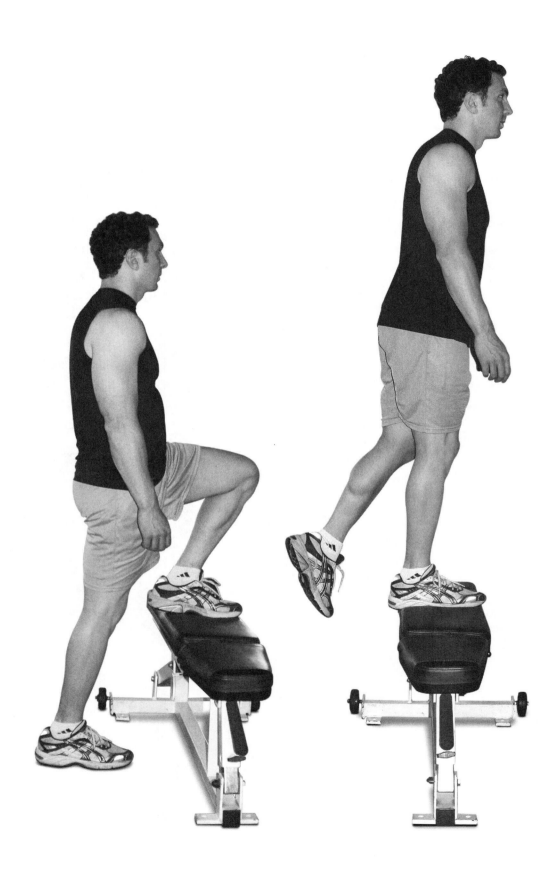

# THE STEP TEST

This simple test is designed to measure your cardiovascular endurance.

## PERFORMING THE STEP TEST

Be sure that you prepare your body by doing a few warmup exercises before engaging in this test (see section on warmup and stretching).

**PROCEDURE:** Before you begin this test, ensure that you have become proficient at checking your pulse rate manually (see section on aerobic exercise in chapter 1).

Find a suitable platform (bench or a similar sized stair or sturdy box) from which to perform this test. It should be approximately 12 inches in height.

Stand tall and keep your back straight and stomach muscles tucked in.

For balance, keep your hands at your side or on your hips.

Step on and off the box for three minutes. Step up with one foot and then the other. Step down with one foot followed by the other foot. Try to maintain a steady four-beat cycle. It's easy to maintain if you say, "up, up, down, down." Go at a steady and consistent pace. Step up on the platform with your entire foot. Be careful not to understep or overstep the platform.

Breathe normally and continuously throughout the test.

At the end of three minutes, remain standing while you immediately check your heart rate. Take your pulse for one minute (e.g., count the total beats from three to four minutes after starting the test).

Compare your results to the table on the next page. Remember, these scores are based on doing the tests as described and may not be accurate if the test is modified at all. This home step test is based loosely on the Canadian Home Fitness Test, and the results below are also based from data collected from performing this test. Don't worry too much about how you rate—just try and improve your own score.

**Your final scores can now be recorded using the chart below:**

| | | |
|---|---|---|
| Excellent/Good | = | scores 3 points |
| Above Average | = | scores 2 points |
| Average/Below Average | = | scores 1 point |
| Below Average | = | scores ½ point |
| Poor/Very Poor | = | scores 0 points |

**Now record your recovery heart rate (RecHR) readings here:**

Date/RecHR:_____

Date/RecHR:_____

Date/RecHR:_____

## HOW WELL DID I DO?

Ratings for both men and women are indicated in the chart below. Simply correspond your age with your final heart rate in the gender related chart below.

## THREE-MINUTE STEP TEST (MEN)

| Age | 18-25 | 26-35 | 36-45 | 46-55 | 56-65 | 65+ |
|---|---|---|---|---|---|---|
| Excellent | <79 | <81 | <83 | <87 | <86 | <88 |
| Good | 79-89 | 81-89 | 83-96 | 87-97 | 86-97 | 88-96 |
| Above Average | 90-99 | 90-99 | 97-103 | 98-105 | 98-103 | 97-103 |
| Average | 100-105 | 100-107 | 104-112 | 106-116 | 104-112 | 104-113 |
| Below Average | 106-116 | 108-117 | 113-119 | 117-122 | 113-120 | 114-120 |
| Poor | 117-128 | 118-128 | 120-130 | 123-132 | 121-129 | 121-130 |
| Very Poor | >128 | >128 | >130 | >132 | >129 | >130 |

## THREE-MINUTE STEP TEST (WOMEN)

| Age | 18-25 | 26-35 | 36-45 | 46-55 | 56-65 | 65+ |
|---|---|---|---|---|---|---|
| Excellent | <85 | <88 | <90 | <94 | <95 | <90 |
| Good | 85-98 | 88-99 | 90-102 | 94-104 | 95-104 | 90-102 |
| Above Average | 99-108 | 100-111 | 103-110 | 105-115 | 105-112 | 103-115 |
| Average | 109-117 | 112-119 | 111-118 | 116-120 | 113-118 | 116-122 |
| Below Average | 118-126 | 120-126 | 119-128 | 121-129 | 119-128 | 123-128 |
| Poor | 127-140 | 127-138 | 129-140 | 130-135 | 129-139 | 129-134 |
| Very Poor | >140 | >138 | >140 | >135 | >139 | >134 |

## MUSCLE ENDURANCE TEST

This component of your personal fitness test aims to identify the overall condition of your strength and endurance by using three key exercises. You'll be using the push-up to test your general upper body condition and the basic sit-up for checking out the condition of your mid-section. To test for lower body condition, you'll finally perform the leg squat.

You should be adequately warmed up from first performing the Aerobic Step Test. If for any reason you feel that your body has cooled down, then re-warm your body by doing some of the simple warmup exercises and stretches described in the warming up and stretching section.

The following tests can often induce the "competitive spirit" in even the most hardened exercise abstainer. It is not a contest, so take my advice and work at a pace that is both comfortable and safe. There is no time limit placed on completing any of these tests. Perform as many repetitions as you feel able to. Once you cease the exercise, then the test is complete. Then note down your result. It's vitally important to maintain good form and technique throughout each exercise. Be sure to breathe normally throughout each exercise. The correct breathing procedure is: breathe out on exertion and in on the return of each exercise.

LET'S START — *Good* LUCK!

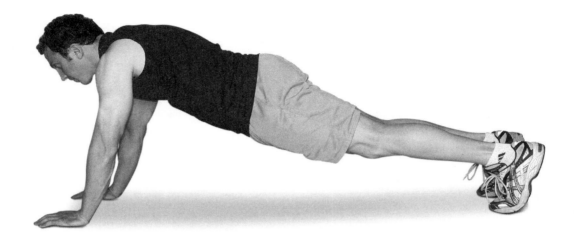

## PUSH-UP TEST:

How many can you do? Men should use the standard "military style" push-up position with only the hands and the toes touching the floor. Women have the additional option of using the "bent knee" position.

Using a mat or padded surface, kneel down, hands on either side of the chest. Keep your back straight and distribute your body weight evenly over your hands and knees/feet. Bend at your elbows to lower your chest to the floor. Finally, extend your arms to return to the start position.

Do as many push-ups as possible until you are reasonably exhausted. Count the total number of push-ups performed. Compare your results to the table below to find out how you rate.

### HOW DID YOU DO?

Remember, these scores are based on doing the tests as described and may not be accurate if the test is modified at all. Again, don't worry too much about how you rate now; the important thing is to improve your scores over time.

## PUSH-UP TEST (MEN)

| Age | 17-19 | 20-29 | 30-39 | 40-49 | 50-59 | 60-65 |
|---|---|---|---|---|---|---|
| Excellent | >56 | >47 | >41 | >34 | >31 | >30 |
| Good | 47-56 | 39-47 | 34-41 | 28-34 | 25-31 | 24-30 |
| Above Average | 35-46 | 30-39 | 25-33 | 21-28 | 18-24 | 17-23 |
| Average | 19-34 | 17-29 | 13-24 | 11-20 | 9-17 | 6-16 |
| Below Average | 11-18 | 10-16 | 8-12 | 6-10 | 5-8 | 3-5 |
| Poor | 4-10 | 4-9 | 2-7 | 1-5 | 1-4 | 1-2 |
| Very Poor | <4 | <4 | <2 | 0 | 0 | 0 |

## PUSH-UP TEST (WOMEN)

| Age | 17-19 | 20-29 | 30-39 | 40-49 | 50-59 | 60-65 |
|---|---|---|---|---|---|---|
| Excellent | >35 | >36 | >37 | >31 | >25 | >23 |
| Good | 27-35 | 30-36 | 30-37 | 25-31 | 21-25 | 19-23 |
| Above Average | 21-27 | 23-29 | 22-30 | 18-24 | 15-20 | 13-18 |
| Average | 11-20 | 12-22 | 10-21 | 8-17 | 7-14 | 5-12 |
| Below Average | 6-10 | 7-11 | 5-9 | 4-7 | 3-6 | 2-4 |
| Poor | 2-5 | 2-6 | 1-4 | 1-3 | 1-2 | 1 |
| Very Poor | 0-1 | 0-1 | 0 | 0 | 0 | 0 |

**Your final scores can now be recorded using the chart above:**

| | | |
|---|---|---|
| Excellent/Good | = | scores 3 points |
| Above Average | = | scores 2 points |
| Average/Below Average | = | scores 1 point |
| Below Average | = | scores ½ point |
| Poor/Very Poor | = | scores 0 points |

**Record your results here:**

Date/Number:_____

Date/Number:_____

Date/Number:_____

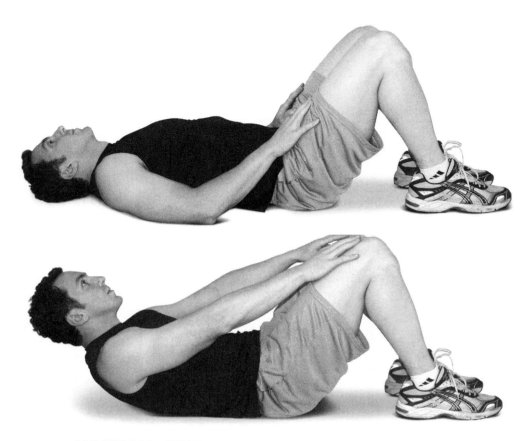

## ABDOMINAL TEST

Abdominal muscle strength and endurance is important for core stability and back support. This sit-up test measures the strength and endurance of the abdominals and hip-flexor muscles. How many sit-ups can you do in one minute? Count how many you can do in one minute and then check the chart below for your rating.

**STARTING POSITION:** Lie on a carpeted or cushioned floor with your knees bent at approximately right angles, with feet flat on the ground. Your hands should be resting on your thighs.

**TECHNIQUE:** Squeeze your stomach, push your back flat into the floor, and raise your torso high enough for your hands to slide along your thighs to touch the tops of your knees. Avoid pulling with your neck or head and keep your lower back on the floor. Then return to the starting position.

## HOW DID YOU DO?

Compare your results to the table below. Remember, these scores are based on doing the tests as described and may not be accurate if the test is modified at all. Don't worry too much about how you rate—just try and improve your own score.

## ONE-MINUTE SIT-UP TEST (MEN)

| Age | 18-25 | 26-35 | 36-45 | 46-55 | 56-65 | 65+ |
|---|---|---|---|---|---|---|
| Excellent | >49 | >45 | >41 | >35 | >31 | >28 |
| Good | 44-49 | 40-45 | 35-41 | 29-35 | 25-31 | 22-28 |
| Above Average | 39-43 | 35-39 | 30-34 | 25-28 | 21-24 | 19-21 |
| Average | 35-38 | 31-34 | 27-29 | 22-24 | 17-20 | 15-18 |
| Below Average | 31-34 | 29-30 | 23-26 | 18-21 | 13-16 | 11-14 |
| Poor | 25-30 | 22-28 | 17-22 | 13-17 | 9-12 | 7-10 |
| Very Poor | <25 | <22 | <17 | <9 | <9 | <7 |

## ONE-MINUTE SIT-UP TEST (WOMEN)

| Age | 18-25 | 26-35 | 36-45 | 46-55 | 56-65 | 65+ |
|---|---|---|---|---|---|---|
| Excellent | >43 | >39 | >33 | >27 | >24 | >23 |
| Good | 37-43 | 33-39 | 27-33 | 22-27 | 18-24 | 17-23 |
| Above Average | 33-36 | 29-32 | 23-26 | 18-21 | 13-17 | 14-16 |
| Average | 29-32 | 25-28 | 19-22 | 14-17 | 10-12 | 11-13 |
| Below Average | 25-28 | 21-24 | 15-18 | 10-13 | 7-9 | 5-10 |
| Poor | 18-24 | 13-20 | 7-14 | 5-9 | 3-6 | 2-4 |
| Very Poor | <18 | <20 | <7 | <5 | <3 | <2 |

## YOUR FINAL SCORES CAN NOW BE RECORDED USING THE CHART BELOW:

| | | |
|---|---|---|
| Excellent/Good | = | scores 3 points |
| Above Average | = | scores 2 points |
| Average/Below Average | = | scores 1 point |
| Below Average | = | scores ½ point |
| Poor/Very Poor | = | scores 0 points |

### Record your results here:

**Date/Number:**_____

Date/Number:_____

Date/Number:_____

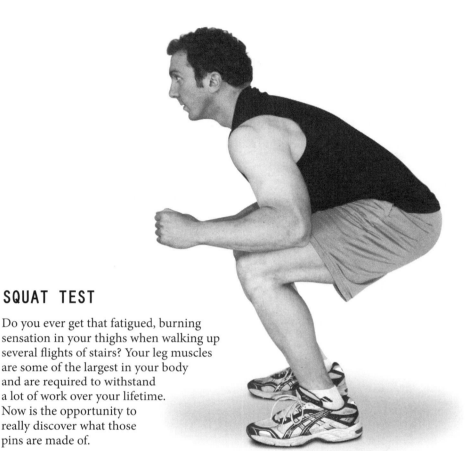

## SQUAT TEST

Do you ever get that fatigued, burning
sensation in your thighs when walking up
several flights of stairs? Your leg muscles
are some of the largest in your body
and are required to withstand
a lot of work over your lifetime.
Now is the opportunity to
really discover what those
pins are made of.

Technique: Stand in front of a chair
or bench with your feet shoulder's width
apart, facing away from it. Place your hands on your hips.
Bend at your knees to lower yourself into a squat position and lean slightly
forward, maintaining a straight back throughout. Lightly touch the chair
before standing back up. Ensure that you do not lock your knees at the top.

An ideal sized chair or bench is one that places your knees at right angles
when you are sitting. Keep doing this for one minute.

Write down how many squats you can do. After you work out for awhile, take
the test again to see how much your lower body strength has improved.

## HOW DID YOU DO?

Compare your results to the table below. Remember, these scores are based
on doing the tests as described and may not be accurate if the test is modified
at all. Don't worry too much about how you rate—just try and improve your
own score.

## SQUAT TEST (MEN)

| Age | 18-25 | 26-35 | 36-45 | 46-55 | 56-65 | 65+ |
|---|---|---|---|---|---|---|
| Excellent | >49 | >45 | >41 | >35 | >31 | >28 |
| Good | 44-49 | 40-45 | 35-41 | 29-35 | 25-31 | 22-28 |
| Above Average | 39-43 | 35-39 | 30-34 | 25-38 | 21-24 | 19-21 |
| Average | 35-38 | 31-34 | 27-29 | 22-24 | 17-20 | 15-18 |
| Below Average | 31-34 | 29-30 | 23-26 | 18-21 | 13-16 | 11-14 |
| Poor | 25-30 | 22-28 | 17-22 | 13-17 | 9-12 | 7-10 |
| Very Poor | <25 | <22 | <17 | <9 | <9 | <7 |

## SQUAT TEST (WOMEN)

| Age | 18-25 | 26-35 | 36-45 | 46-55 | 56-65 | 65+ |
|---|---|---|---|---|---|---|
| Excellent | >43 | >39 | >33 | >27 | >24 | >23 |
| Good | 37-43 | 33-39 | 27-33 | 22-27 | 18-24 | 17-23 |
| Above Average | 33-36 | 29-32 | 23-26 | 18-21 | 13-17 | 14-16 |
| Average | 29-32 | 25-28 | 19-22 | 14-17 | 10-12 | 11-13 |
| Below Average | 25-28 | 21-24 | 15-18 | 10-13 | 7-9 | 5-10 |
| Poor | 18-24 | 13-20 | 7-14 | 5-9 | 3-6 | 2-4 |
| Very Poor | <18 | <20 | <7 | <5 | <3 | <2 |

**Your final scores can now be recorded using the chart below:**

| | | |
|---|---|---|
| Excellent/Good | = | scores 3 points |
| Above Average | = | scores 2 points |
| Average/Below Average | = | scores 1 point |
| Below Average | = | scores ½ point |
| Poor/Very Poor | = | scores 0 points |

**Record your results here:**

Date/Number:_____

Date/Number:_____

Date/Number:_____

**Now add up your total scores for all tests and make a note below**


Total Score:_____


If you scored the maximum points of 46, then your rating is high and your suitability for exercising gets the green light. After having completed the fitness test, I recommend that you choose the Specialist Exerciser plan.

If you scored more than 31, then your rating is good. After having completed the fitness test, you'll probably progress quite rapidly in the Adventurous Exerciser plan.

If you scored between 16 and 30, this suggests that you should be taking stock of your current physical condition and start by using either the Exercise Neophyte or Progressive Exerciser plan.

If you scored 15 or below, then you may be at risk for participating in exercise. Seek your doctor's advice before you start the fitness test.


## RETESTING

To evaluate and monitor your progress, I advise that you undergo the fitness test periodically. You should make a note of all of your results and draw a comparison between your initial test and the current one. By doing so, you can gauge how well you are doing, and it will help you to identify areas of your strengths and weaknesses. This, in turn, will enable you to fine-tune your exercise program and address any deficiencies. After your eight-week retest, you may find that testing yourself every three months is more than adequate.

# CHAPTER *Five:*

## GYM, WHAT GYM?

CHAPTER FIVE:

# GYM, WHAT *gym?*

## GET ULTRA-TONED AND LEAN WITH THE CELEBRITY BODY ON A BUDGET 'NO GYM REQUIRED' WORKOUTS!

The *Celebrity Body on a Budget* structured workouts are a perfect fusion of potent cardiovascular and resistance training designed to be easy to follow, give you a great workout, target fat loss, build muscle tone and strength, and improve cardiovascular fitness. Let's not forget about the built-in benefit of following your own low-cost exercise program—remaining faithful to the ethos of this book!

You can choose your own personally tailored workouts from a varied selection of "No Gym Required"-style exercise programs that match your current fitness level. There are exercise plans to suit all ages and fitness goals. The four exercise plans are **Exercise Neophyte**, **Progressive Exerciser**, **Adventurous Exerciser**, and **Specialist Exerciser**. With each workout, you'll face a challenge. Each workout is efficient and effective because you work your entire body, simply by going from one exercise to another with limited or no rest

The attractive feature of these workout plans is that little or no equipment is necessary. Your body was meant to move itself around efficiently under a wide variety of circumstances. Using only the weight of your own body as resistance, you will develop an even greater ability to push, jump, land, squat, lunge, reach, twist, and bend. The exercises are fun, yet effective and safe—plus they lead to realistic results. These workouts involve calisthenics such as push-ups, various squats, jumping jacks, abdominal crunches, and other body weight exercises. In some instances, some basic and minimal equipment such as a wall, a chair, a bench, or a small selection of weights will be necessary to complete your exercise routine. The difference between these exercise programs and others lies in the variety they offer over continuous, solo activity exercise such as running, rowing, and cycling.

With *Celebrity Body on a Budget*, your challenge is to take your body to its limit in a safe and enjoyable manner. You work, you sweat, and, best of all, you burn calories like a furnace, resulting in a fitter, stronger, and leaner you. These fun and rewarding workouts are designed to keep you motivated and inspired to help fulfill your fitness potential.

## LET'S ANALYZE SOME OF THE MAJOR BENEFITS OF THE CELEBRITY BODY ON A BUDGET EXERCISE PLAN OVER A TRADITIONAL GYM WORKOUT IN MORE DETAIL:

This book's exercises are tremendously versatile. They can be done anywhere and anytime—indoors or outdoors. No matter where you are—you will have an effective physical training method at your disposal! They're easy to fit into a busy schedule—you can do them anywhere at anytime with little equipment. If the weather's nice and you want to enjoy the outdoors, just locate an open patch of ground and you are ready to go. What if it's too cold or raining? Stay inside and improve yourself with these body weight style routines. On a vacation and the hotel doesn't have a gym? No problem, your hotel room will become your new workout environment.

The beauty of the *Celebrity Body on a Budget* workouts is that whenever you want an efficient workout you can have one. The exercises are easy and less complicated, ensuring that you experience a feeling of accomplishment after each session. There are no time restrictions on when you can and when you can't workout. After all, unlike the gym, your body never closes (unless, of course, when it's resting).

These workouts are efficient, helping you work every muscle in your body in a short period of time thus enhancing overall physical fitness. The pace of the exercise schedule helps burn more calories and fat in a short span of time.

Want to start your morning off with a quick, energizing workout using just your own body weight? Jump right in. After a hard day at the office, why not de-stress with a workout and a warm shower before heading for a good night's rest?

These workouts stimulate all the muscles in the body as well as your heart and lungs, providing for the perfect environment in which to burn calories and fat! Not only can these circuits make you stronger, they can simultaneously improve heart and lung power while burning fat. And don't forget the fun factor—with different exercises included, circuit training acts as a psychological booster and is a challenging experience for you. Each exercise is different so you don't get bored with exercise repetition.

These exercises are adaptable to suit your fitness level. The programs are both flexible and modifiable. They are able to be adapted from the beginner level to the serious exerciser level. Your body is made to move in all directions—up, down, forward, backwards, sideways, twisting, bending, etc. This book's workouts use natural movement patterns to improve your own natural movement, therefore improving health, fitness, and shape! You can make them as challenging as you want them to be.

These exercises develop the foundation for other exercise methods and, therefore, are an integral part of any training plan. You will learn and improve the movement of your body. This will allow you to then introduce other training disciplines and equipment into the plan. Once you graduate to employing other training methods, you can choose to maintain your current *Celebrity Body on a Budget* program as a part of your overall fitness training plan to optimize the effectiveness of your body.

In a nutshell, if you have a functional body, you have your very own working gym!

## HOW TO USE YOUR CELEBRITY BODY ON A BUDGET WORKOUT

This section of the book outlines how to structure your own tailor-made training program for general fitness (Exercise Neophyte and Progressive Exerciser programs) or to build on what you have while throwing in a measure of specific performance training (Adventurous Exerciser and Specialist Exerciser programs).

*Celebrity Body on a Budget* workouts consist of a series of exercises performed in succession with minimal rest intervals in between. Due to the quick pace of the exercises, they include exercises that work on all areas of fitness including endurance, strength, flexibility, fat loss, agility, and, best of all, they require little to no equipment. They burn fat, boost weight loss, and result in ultimate fitness. This makes them intense, challenging, and a whole lot of fun. Since you change from one exercise directly into another exercise, your body is getting a complete workout. You'll work out in a shorter time period while still burning tons of calories, plus you'll never get bored, which means you'll feel motivated to work harder and get great results.

To ensure good form and gain an understanding of how to perform each exercise, first look at and study each exercise in your circuit. You may decide to give each one a "dummy run." If you do, be sure to warm up first. Once you are confident in performing each exercise, then it's time for the "real thing." The tempo of each exercise is as crucial as good form, so work at a steady and controlled pace. Move to the next exercise smoothly, but quickly. Avoid rushing your circuit; focus on proper form and making sure that you're not bouncing on the way down or up. If an exercise becomes difficult to complete, then pause for a short time. Sacrificing good form can lead to injury and setbacks in your fitness crusade. Circuit training can be completed two to four times per week. As with resistance training, give yourself at least forty-eight hours between sessions that work the same muscle groups.

# REPETITIONS AND CIRCUITS

Each workout follows in a logical sequence with easy-to-follow exercises so you can make a swift transition from one exercise to the next.

A repetition (or rep) is one complete, single movement of a particular exercise. A circuit represents one completion of all prescribed exercises in the program. When one circuit is complete, you start at the first exercise again for another circuit. Traditionally, the time between exercises in the circuit is short, often moving swiftly on to the next exercise.

You will find that the Exercise Neophyte program has only nine exercises, the Progressive Exerciser comprises twelve exercises, the Adventurous Exerciser includes seventeen exercises, and the Specialist Exerciser program consists of a mouth-watering eighteen exercises.

Each exercise will target different muscle groups from your chest, back, abs, core, arms, and buttocks to thighs and calves. The exercises involving leg movement such as step-ups and lunges are designed to raise the cardiovascular intensity, while the standing weights exercises and abs work allow some comparative interval rest while focusing on muscle conditioning.

By following your workout of three circuits at the prescribed intensity plus warmup and cool down, you should expend in the region of 400 to 600 calories (depending on the program undertaken). That is truly incredible considering you get cardiovascular combined with muscle work, at the same time, and in under an hour of activity.

# SOME CONSIDERATIONS

1. It's imperative that you maintain good form with each lift. Lifts should not be done so fast that you lose form and concentration in the target muscles.

2. Each workout features elements of high-intensity aerobics combined with muscle conditioning. If you can't reach the suggested number of repetitions for any particular exercise, reduce the number while maintaining the pace. For example, perform 12 reps of squats instead of 16 reps and so on.

**3.** To make sure you are exercising in a safe zone, particularly if you are unfit or have a medical condition, use a heart rate monitor or manual pulse check to keep track of the intensity. Bear in mind that these workouts are designed to raise your heart rate to the point where you are breathing "somewhat hard." If you don't bother with heart rate monitoring, combine the training heart rate zone with the talk test. The talk test implies that you are able to converse adequately, if not altogether comfortably, while exercising. You should never feel completely breathless and unable to talk when engaged in your exercises. If necessary, take a slight pause between each exercise or do fewer repetitions and move more slowly between exercises. You can opt to have a brief water break between each circuit.

**4.** Beforehand, choose a set of dumbbells. It's important to keep the weights heavy enough for you to complete the maximum number of repetitions of each weighted exercise, which means you can't do more than the indicated number of reps without your good form failing. Try to avoid reducing the dumbbell weight during your workout, as these weights should be heavy enough to build strength and muscle conditioning. The lower body exercises, such as the weighted lunges and squats, are done with the same dumbbells.

**5.** Use each exercise to work your abdominals. Although not every exercise targets the abdominals directly, remember to pull your abs into the brace position in preparation for each lift or movement.

**6.** These workouts can be done at home, at a gym, or in the park four or five times in a week, but my recommendation is to do no more than three sessions. You should supplement your circuits with at least one pure cardio session such as running, power walking, or swimming plus at least one pure resistance training day with weights.

---

**EQUIPMENT REQUIREMENTS FOR YOUR CIRCUIT:**

1. Step platform or equivalent of at least 8 inches in height.

2. a) Pair of dumbbells or bottles of water *(see notes re: selecting correct weight further on)* or b) strength bands.

3. Jump/skipping rope.

4. Exercise mat or thick towels or rug.

5. Water to drink!

# WARMING UP AND COOLING DOWN

## WARMING UP

Your body is more efficient when it is warmed up and less likely to suffer damage. The goal of the warmup is to get your blood circulating and your body temperature rising in order to prepare for higher intensity exercise.

Therefore, it's vital to warm up as a prelude to more vigorous exercise. It should take place before you embark on your workout. Layers of warm clothing should be worn if you are in a cold environment. You can then strip back the layers once you feel adequately warm.

## BENEFITS OF WARMING UP

·   Prepares your body for exercise by increasing circulation and delivering more oxygen to the muscles.

·   Raises body temperature so your body is more efficient and less likely to suffer damage during strenuous exercise.

·   Increases the heart rate in readiness for more strenuous exercise.

·   Mobilizes joints so they move more freely and are less likely to be damaged.

Start with a light warmup of about ten minutes. Gradually increase the pace or intensity of the warmup activity over a period of a few minutes. It may be a good idea to add in some stretching, although there is much debate as to the importance or usefulness of pre-exercise stretching. I am personally of the opinion that if you have the time, then it's wise to perform the stretches, particularly those of your major working muscles. However, as part of your cool down, it is imperative that you conclude your workout with stretching.

## SUGGESTED WARMUP EXERCISES

·   Light marching on the spot
    *(more suited to Neophyte and Progressive program).*

·   Light jogging on the spot
    *(more suited to Neophyte and Progressive program).*

·   Brisk walking up stairs several times *(suitable for all programs).*

·   Light skipping with or without rope
    *(more suited to Adventurous and Specialist program).*

·   If you have access to equipment, spend time warming up
    on your piece of equipment *(suitable for all programs).*

## COOL DOWN

The cool down is the part a lot of people forget. In fact, reasons for cooling down are stronger than those for warming up. It is vital to allow the body to return to its pre-exercise state. In effect, the cool down phase of your workout will be more or less identical to your warmup phase. The main difference is that the intensity of your cool down should be lower.

Therefore, cooling down should consist of five to ten minutes of light-intensity exercises. Any activity will suffice. Your heart rate and body temperature should decrease over this period.

Five to ten minutes of static stretching exercises should follow.

Stretches are more appropriate to the cool down because they help muscles to relax, realign muscle fibers, and re-establish their normal range of movement. These stretches should be held for a minimum of fifteen seconds each—longer if you can spare the time. You may wish to be protected against rapid cooling of the skin, by wearing warm, loose clothing.

## BENEFITS OF A COOL DOWN

- Allows the heart rate to return to its resting rate.

- Dissipates muscle lactate, a product of high-intensity exercise.

- Prevents "delayed onset muscle soreness" (DOMS) the next day.

- Reduces the chances of dizziness or fainting caused by the pooling of venous blood at the extremities.

- Replenishes fuel supplies in the muscles.

- Increases suppleness.

# SUGGESTED STATIC STRETCHES

### SHOULDER STRETCH

Stand with your feet slightly apart, tummy tight, and knees slightly bent. Raise your arms above your head, rotating your wrists and place your palms together. Straighten your arms as much as comfortable until you feel an adequate stretch directly in your shoulders. Hold for 15-30 seconds.

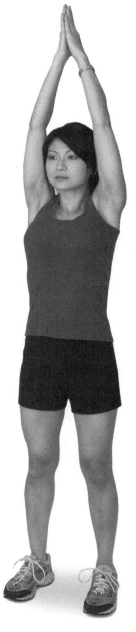

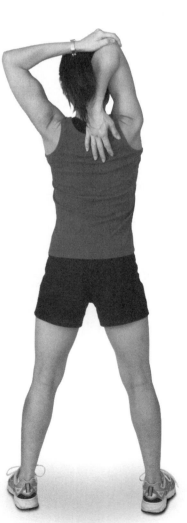

### UPPER ARM STRETCH

Stand with your feet slightly apart, tummy tight, and knees slightly bent. Raise one arm and place the hand of that arm between your shoulder blades. Place your free hand on the elbow of the arm being stretched. Gently ease the elbow behind your head until you feel a positive stretch. Hold for 15-30 seconds. Change sides when complete.

## OUTER SHOULDER STRETCH

While standing, place one arm across your chest and cup the hand of your free arm over the elbow of the arm being stretched. Apply gentle pressure with your hand to the elbow until you feel a positive, pain-free stretch in your outer shoulder. Hold for 15-30 seconds. Change sides when complete.

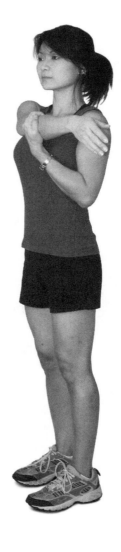

## CHEST STRETCH

While standing, take both hands behind your back, linking your fingers together with your palms turned in. Gently raise your arms away from your body, simultaneously bringing your shoulder blades together and easing your chest forward until a positive stretch is felt in your chest region. Hold for 15-30 seconds.

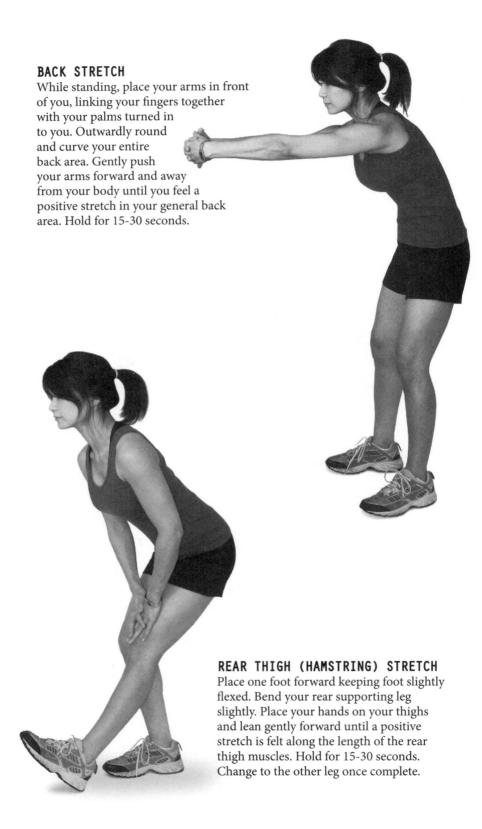

## BACK STRETCH

While standing, place your arms in front of you, linking your fingers together with your palms turned in to you. Outwardly round and curve your entire back area. Gently push your arms forward and away from your body until you feel a positive stretch in your general back area. Hold for 15-30 seconds.

## REAR THIGH (HAMSTRING) STRETCH

Place one foot forward keeping foot slightly flexed. Bend your rear supporting leg slightly. Place your hands on your thighs and lean gently forward until a positive stretch is felt along the length of the rear thigh muscles. Hold for 15-30 seconds. Change to the other leg once complete.

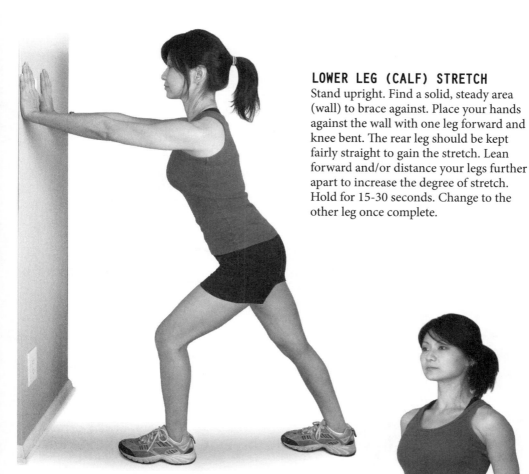

## LOWER LEG (CALF) STRETCH

Stand upright. Find a solid, steady area (wall) to brace against. Place your hands against the wall with one leg forward and knee bent. The rear leg should be kept fairly straight to gain the stretch. Lean forward and/or distance your legs further apart to increase the degree of stretch. Hold for 15-30 seconds. Change to the other leg once complete.

## FRONT THIGH (QUADRICEP) STRETCH

Stand upright. For support, hold onto a steady surface. Slightly bend your supporting leg. Raise the other leg up and grasp your ankle, gently bringing your heel up toward your buttock. Gently push your hips forward and ease the leg backwards to gain a positive stretch. Hold for 15-30 seconds. Change to the other leg once complete.

Now that you've got a grip on the warmup and cool down exercises, it's time to commence a full structured workout. Complete all exercises for your program rhythmically and continuously without stopping for the allotted time or number of repetitions. All exercises should be performed in a controlled manner while emphasizing good form. Breathing on a regular basis is also vitally important. This is often overlooked, particularly by newcomers to exercise as they tend to forget to breathe and wonder why they feel like passing out.

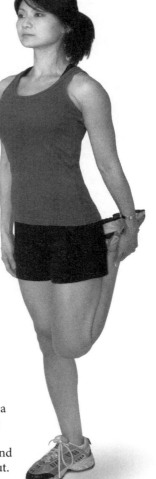

# EXERCISE NEOPHYTE PROGRAM

Begin with 2 circuits and 10 repetitions for each of the exercises described below. Perform this routine 3 times a week on non-consecutive days for six weeks. Consult the chart below for a weekly progress plan. The numbers in the chart suggest the amount of circuits followed by the amount of repetitions you should perform. After completing the sixth week of this program, move onto the Progressive Exerciser Program.

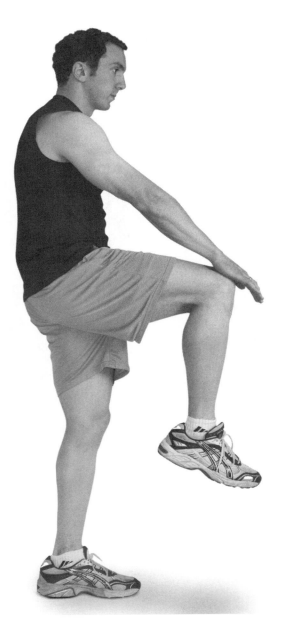

|  | Circuit x Reps |
|---|---|
| Week 1 | 2 x 10 |
| Week 2 | 2 x 12 |
| Week 3 | 2 x 14 |
| Week 4 | 2 x16 |
| Week 5 | 3 x 10 |
| Week 6 | 3 x 12 |

## MARCHING KNEE-UPS

Start by marching on the spot with high knee lift. Place your hand outward at waist height. Pick your knees up to waist height and pump your legs alternatively so knees touch hands. Speed of movements and/or height of knees controls degree of effort used.

## MODIFIED PUSH-UPS

Begin in the all-fours position on the floor. Place hands slightly wider than shoulder width apart. Keep your hands and knees in contact with the ground. Keep the tummy tucked and the back straight. Bend your arms and lower your chest to the floor. Then push your body upward as you extend your arms, returning to the front-support position.

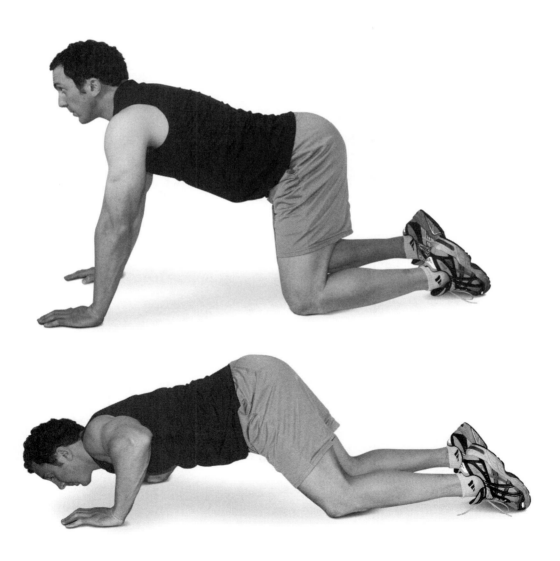

## ABDOMINAL CRUNCHES

Lie on your back with your knees bent and feet flat on the floor. Place your fingertips to the side of your head just behind your ears. Push your lower back into the floor flattening the arch and hold. Curl up slowly so both your shoulders lift off the floor a few inches. Hold for a count of 2 and return to the start position. Keep your head up and avoid tucking your chin to your chest.

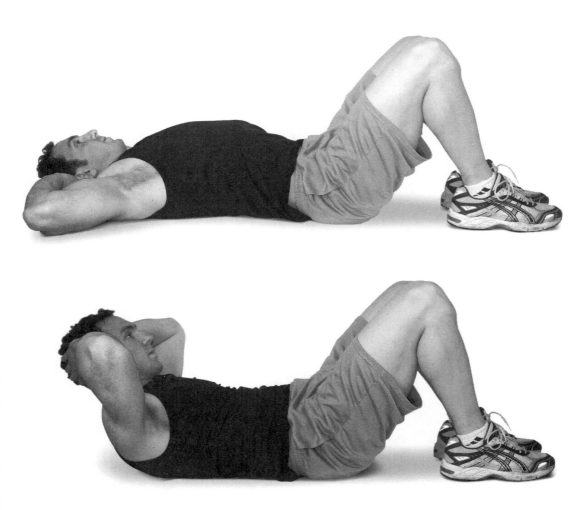

## WALL SQUAT THRUSTS

Lean into a wall with your hands and keep your feet shoulder width apart several feet from the wall. Slowly jump forward with both legs about 18 inches away from the wall. Slowly jump back again to the start position. Continue jumping back and forth. As you improve your fitness, increase your back/forth leg jump speed.

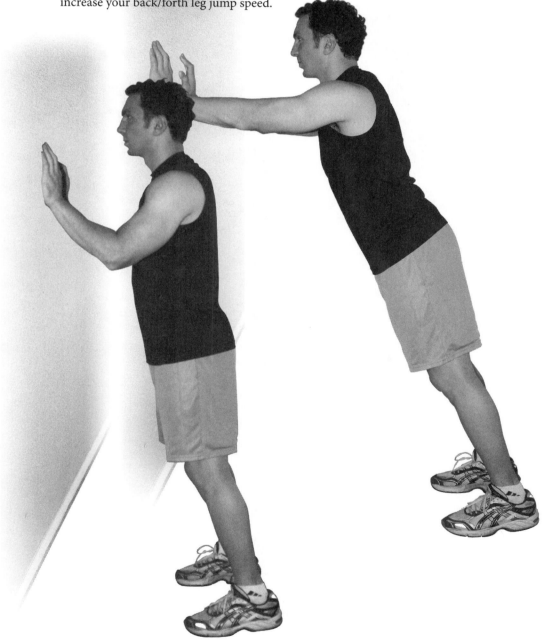

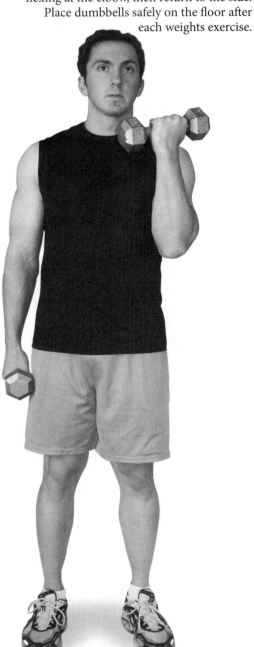

## DUMBBELL CURLS

Hold the dumbbells at your sides, palms facing inward (like a hammer grip). Do 12 alternate curls with each arm lifting the dumbbell to the shoulder by rotating the forearm so that the palms face upward, flexing at the elbow, then return to the side. Place dumbbells safely on the floor after each weights exercise.

## SIT-UPS WITH TWIST

Lie back onto the floor with knees bent and hands behind ears. Keep elbows back. Head should be in a neutral position with a space between chin and chest. Leading with the chin and chest toward the ceiling, contract the abdominals and raise shoulders off floor. As you come up, twist one shoulder toward the opposite knee. Return to start position and repeat with the other shoulder.

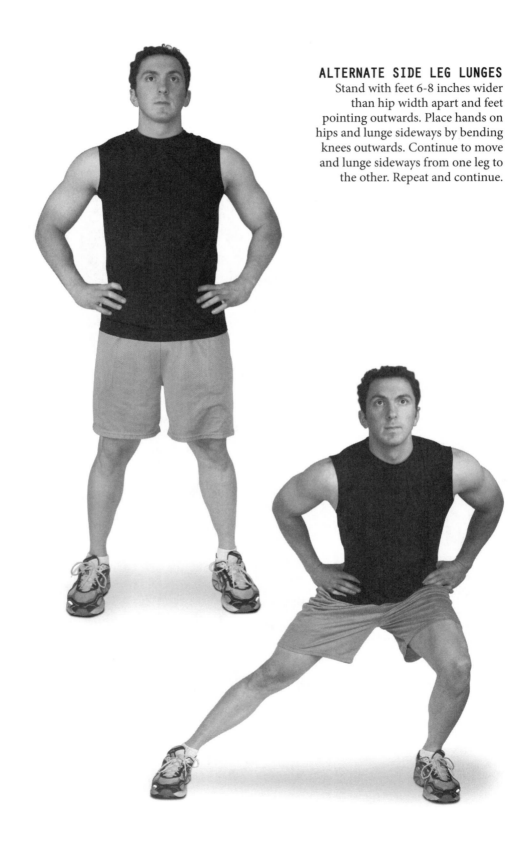

## ALTERNATE SIDE LEG LUNGES

Stand with feet 6-8 inches wider than hip width apart and feet pointing outwards. Place hands on hips and lunge sideways by bending knees outwards. Continue to move and lunge sideways from one leg to the other. Repeat and continue.

## BENCH DIPS

Sit upright on the edge of a sturdy bench and place hands hip width apart, palms down and gripping the edge of the bench. Place legs in front of you and bend knees making a right angle. Keep feet flat on the floor. Slide your buttocks off the bench with elbows slightly bent. Allow your body to descend to the floor by bending at the elbows until the elbows are at 90-degree angle. Extend up again to return to start position.

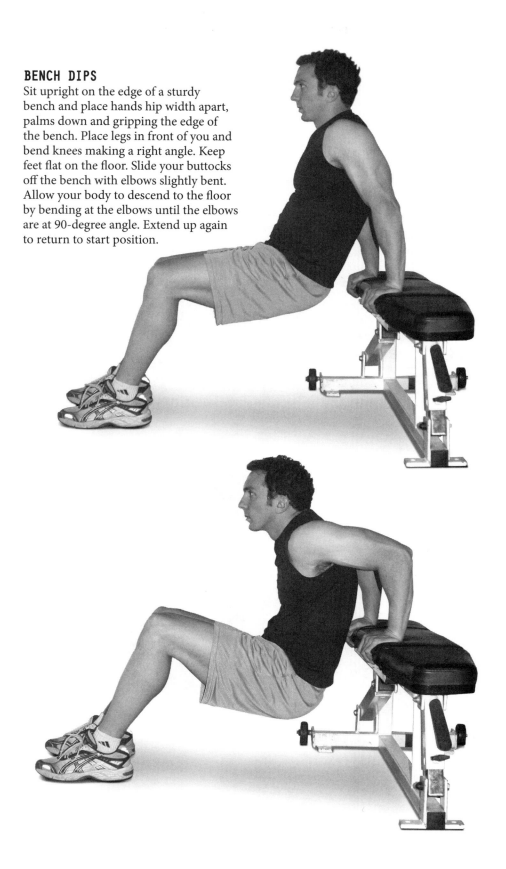

## MUMMY CRUNCHES

Lie on your back with knees bent and feet flat on floor. Place and fold arms across the chest. Keep a small gap between chin and chest. As you curl shoulders off the floor, brace the tummy muscles by drawing them in. To return, lower shoulders to floor and continue.

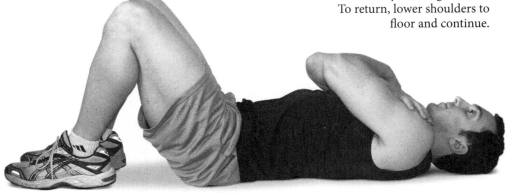

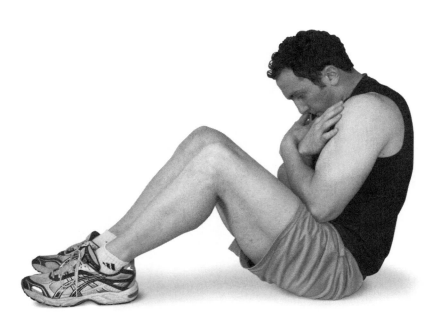

# PROGRESSIVE EXERCISER PROGRAM

Begin with 2 circuits and 10 repetitions for each of the exercises described below. Perform this routine 3 times a week on non-consecutive days. Consult the chart below for a weekly progress plan. The numbers in the chart suggest the amount of circuits followed by the amount of repetitions you should perform. After completing the tenth week of this program, move onto the Adventurous Exerciser Program.

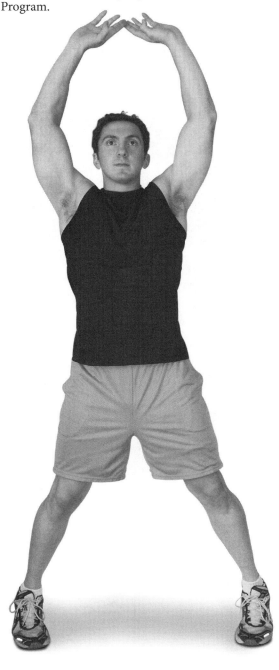

|         | Circuit x Reps |
|---------|----------------|
| Week 1  | 2 x 10         |
| Week 2  | 2 x 12         |
| Week 3  | 2 x 14         |
| Week 4  | 2 x 16         |
| Week 5  | 3 x 10         |
| Week 6  | 3 x 12         |
| Week 7  | 3 x 14         |
| Week 8  | 3 x 16         |
| Week 9  | 3 x 18         |
| Week 10 | 3 x 20         |

## JUMPING JACKS

Start with your legs together and your arms by your side. In one motion, jump and spread your legs out to the side while your arms sweep out and up over your head. Land in this position and then return to the starting position and repeat.

Hold dumbbells horizontally at the shoulders with upright arms, palms facing up. Lift the dumbbells overhead with full arm extension making sure not to lock the elbows out explosively. Return to the shoulder and immediately repeat the exercise.

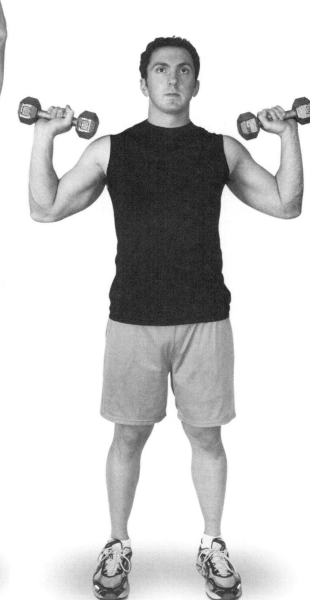

## BACKWARD STRIDE

Stand with feet together. Stride backward with one leg by bending the knee to a right angle while raising the arms to shoulder level. Lower the arms to your side and repeat with the other leg. Continue by alternating legs.

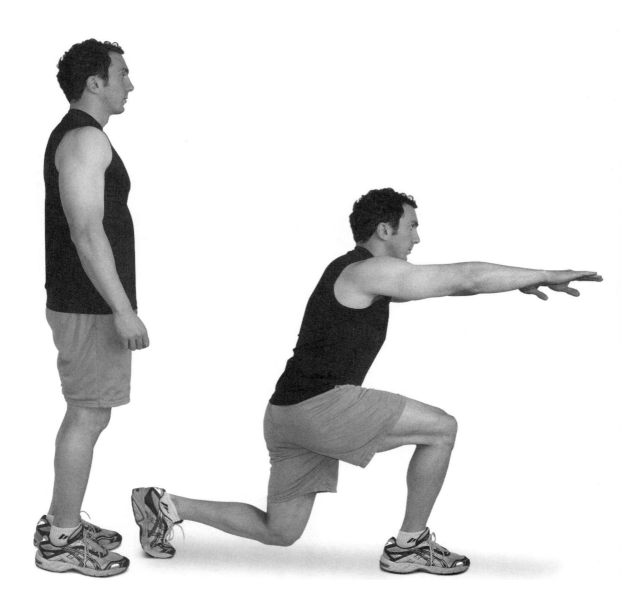

## REVERSE CRUNCH

Lie on your back with your hands out to your sides, head kept back and bend your knees. Bring your knees toward your chest until your hips come up slightly off the floor (avoid rocking). Keep the knees together in a fixed position and imagine bringing your belly button toward your spine as you curl knees to chest. Hold and squeeze abs for one second and repeat for the prescribed number of repetitions/time.

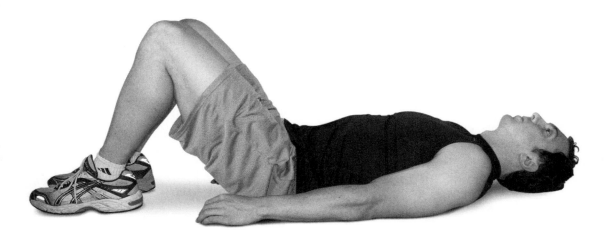

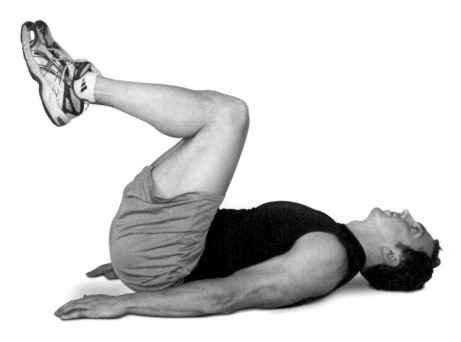

## DUMBBELL SQUATS

Hold dumbbells at the sides with arms long. Squat down, bending at the knee until thighs are approximately parallel with the floor ensuring the knees are not extended too far beyond the toes. The back should be kept straight or slightly arched inward, the neutral position, but not rounded at the shoulders or spine, with head still, looking forward. Straighten to the starting position and repeat the squat.

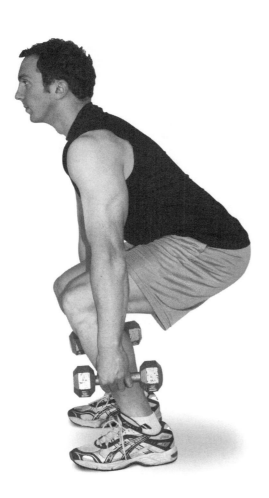
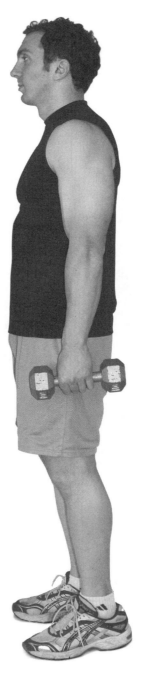

## BENT OVER ROWING

Stand with legs hip width apart and knees slightly soft, bend body at waist to lean torso forward. Keep tummy muscles tight and back straight. Hold a dumbbell in each hand hanging down toward the floor with arms extended. Lift dumbbells up toward your shoulders, by bending the elbows past level of body. Return to arms extended position and repeat.

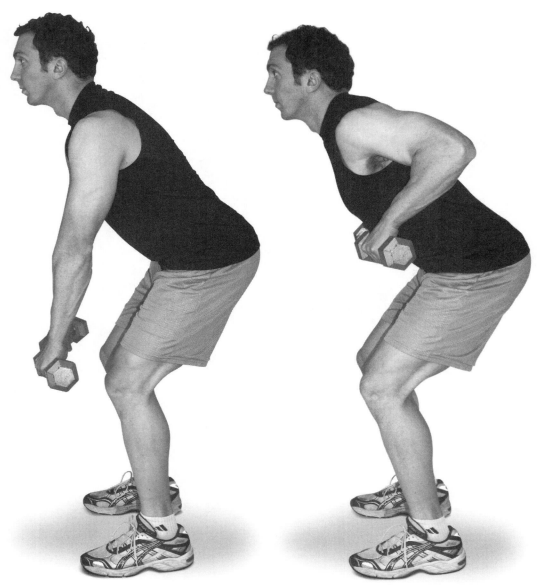

## DOUBLE CRUNCHES

Lie back onto the floor with hands behind ears and knees bent at 90 degrees. Keep elbows back and arms flared out. Head should be in a neutral position with a space between chin and chest. Leading with the chin and chest toward the ceiling, contract the abdominals and raise shoulders off the floor. During the crunch, also bring the knees toward the chest. Return to the start position and repeat.

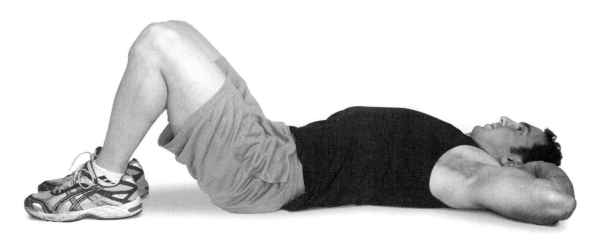

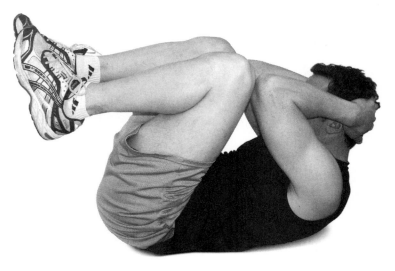

## RICOCHETS

Stand with your feet together and arms by your sides. Keeping your feet together, jump forward a foot or so. Jump back to the starting position. Jump to your left and back to the start, then to the right and back to the start, and then behind you and back to the start. Repeat this sequence by keeping ground contact time minimal and feet together.

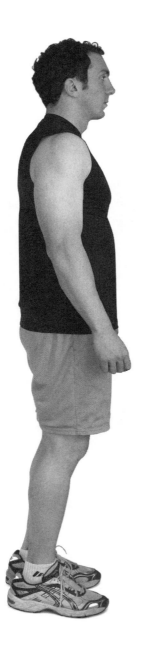
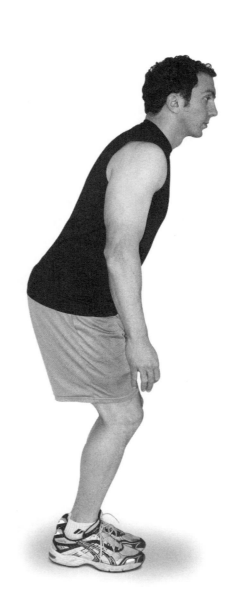

## SUPERMANS

Lie on your stomach with your hands extended above your head and your feet kept together. Slowly raise your arms and legs off the ground a few inches, hold 2 seconds, and then lower. Avoid raising the head and legs beyond 8-12 inches, as excessive hyperextension may cause injury. Repeat for the prescribed number of repetitions/time.

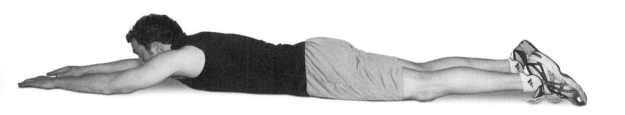

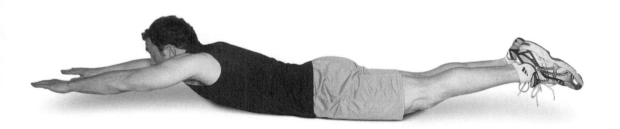

## MODIFIED WIDE PUSH-UPS

Begin in the all-fours position on the floor. Place your hands 4 inches wider than shoulder width apart. Keep your hands and knees in contact with the ground. Keep the tummy tucked and the back straight. Bend your arms and lower your chest to the floor. Then push your body upward as you extend your arms, returning to the front-support position for repeating.

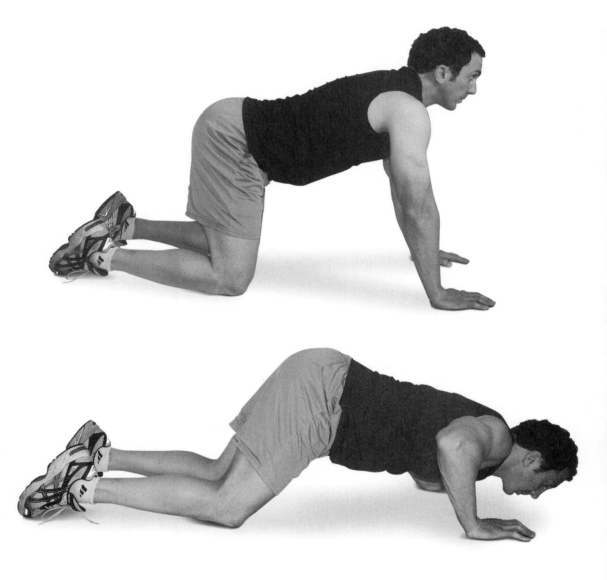

## ALTERNATE FORWARD LUNGES WITH BICEPS CURLS

Start by standing with your feet shoulder width apart and holding a dumbbell in each hand. Step forward with one foot and bend your knees into a lunged position as you curl both dumbbells toward your shoulders. Your back knee should come close to touching the ground (6 inches away), and your front leg should be bent to about 90 degrees at the knee. Maintain your upright posture throughout the movement. Return to the starting position and repeat on the opposite leg.

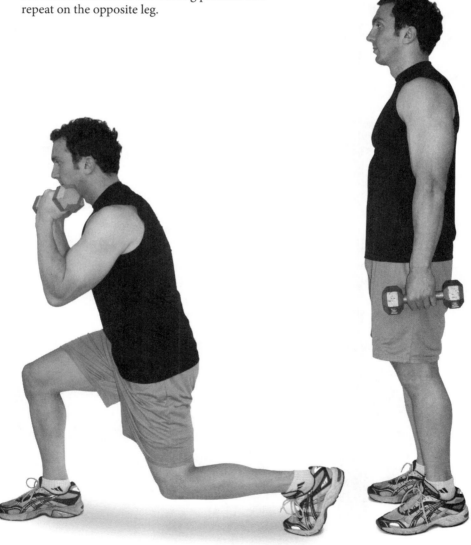

## BICYCLE KICKS

Lie on your back with your knees at chest level and your hands supporting head. Raise and keep the head and shoulder off the floor. Create a subtle twisting action with your upper body as your elbow meets your opposite knee. Alternate this movement. Make sure you keep your back flat during the movement. If you are unable to keep your back flat, then reduce the extension of your legs. Continue to repeat this process as if you were riding a bicycle.

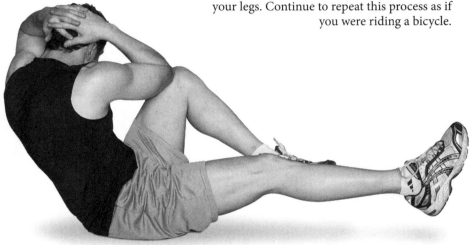

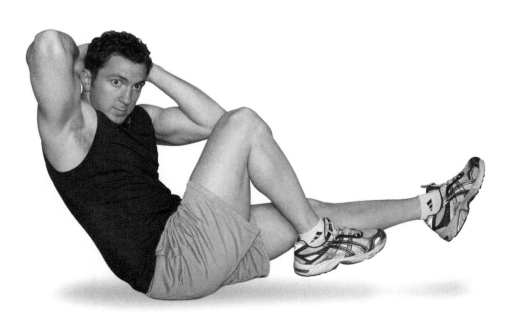

# ADVENTUROUS EXERCISER PROGRAM

Begin with 3 circuits and 12 repetitions for each exercise. Perform this routine
3 times a week on non-consecutive days. Consult the chart below for a weekly
progress plan. The numbers in the chart suggest the amount of circuits
followed by the amount of repetitions you should perform. After completing
the eighth week of this program, move onto the Specialist Exerciser Program.

## DYNAMIC STEP-UPS

Step up onto the step bench starting with the right foot,
follow with the left, then step down with the left and
follow with the right. Alternate the starting foot at half
way if you wish. This exercise should be performed at a
fast pace with good balance and safety. Ensure the step
is anchored safely and solidly before starting. Continue
for a set amount of time/repetitions.

|        | Circuit x Reps |
|--------|----------------|
| Week 1 | 3 x 12 |
| Week 2 | 3 x 14 |
| Week 3 | 3 x 16 |
| Week 4 | 3 x 18 |
| Week 5 | 3 x 20 |
| Week 6 | 3 x 22 |
| Week 7 | 3 x 24 |
| Week 8 | 3 x 26 |

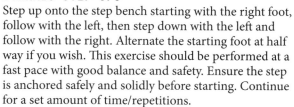

## SIDE JUMPS

Stand with feet together. Jump to the right several feet, thinking of jumping laterally rather than vertically. Keep knees bent and land in a squat position. Land with knees soft and immediately jump back to the left. Continue jumping from side to side. Use a small object to jump over if you like (e.g., a book or broomstick). Repeat for a set amount of time/repetitions.

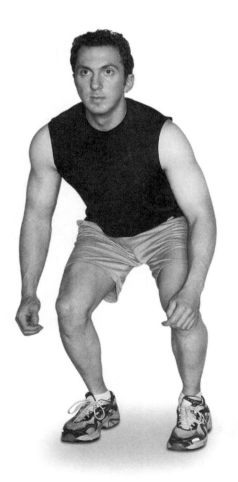

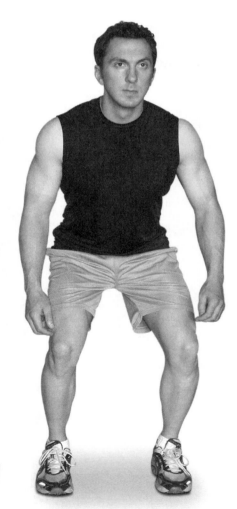

## DIAMOND PUSH-UPS

Begin in the all-fours position on the floor. Place your hands together and make a diamond shape with your thumbs and forefingers. Keep your hands and knees in contact with the ground. Keep your tummy tucked and back straight. Bend your arms and lower your chest to the floor. Then push your body upward as you extend your arms, returning to the start position for repeating. Continue for the prescribed number of repetitions/time.

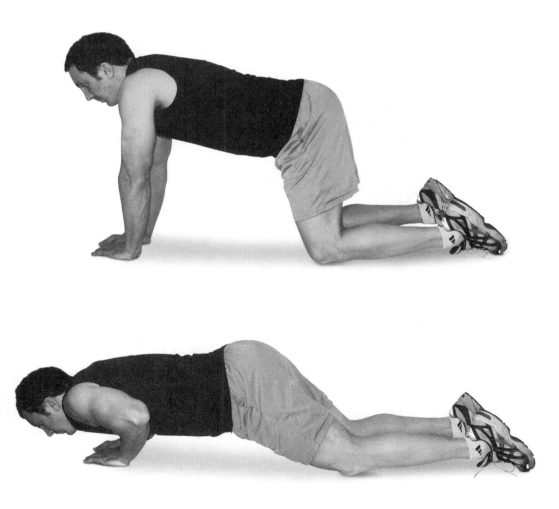

## OBLIQUE CRUNCHES

Lie on your back and place your left foot over your right knee and place your hands behind your ears. Lift your shoulders up off the ground and twist so that your right elbow touches your left knee. Return to the starting position and repeat according to the required repetitions/time. Repeat with the other side—left elbow to right knee.

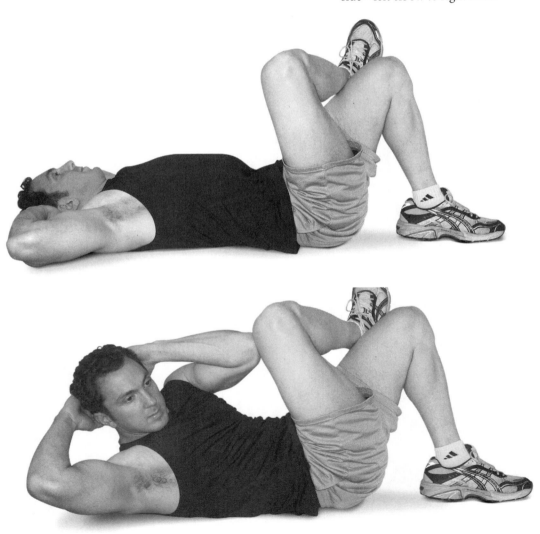

## ONE LEG BALANCE SQUAT AND REACH

Place an object on the floor, several feet in front of you (e.g., a book). Stand on one leg and hold the position steady for 5 seconds. Then slowly squat down, reach out with one arm, and touch the object. Steadily return to an upright position. Stay on one leg at all times. Repeat on the other leg after the set amount of time/repetitions.

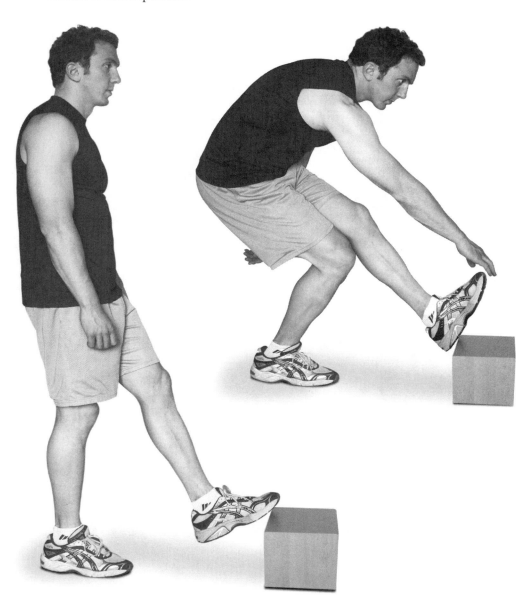

## TREADMILLS

Start in the all-fours position on the floor then extend your legs straight behind you. Bring one knee into your chest, then quickly switch to bring the other knee into your chest. Continue to alternate your feet. Keep stomach muscles tight and back straight and not arched. The action should be a smooth running motion with your arms in a fixed position. Continue.

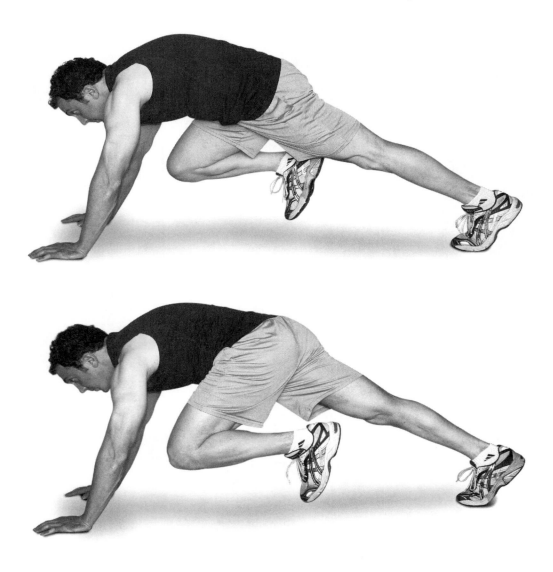

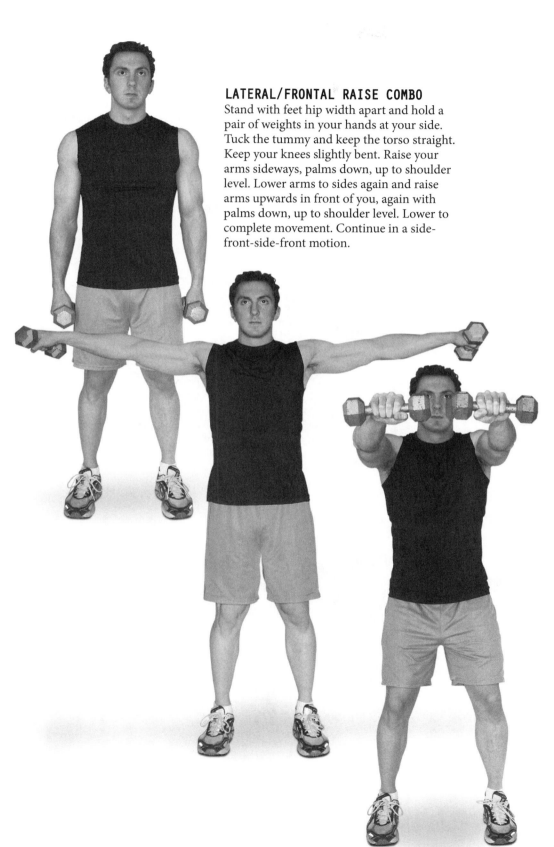

## LATERAL/FRONTAL RAISE COMBO

Stand with feet hip width apart and hold a pair of weights in your hands at your side. Tuck the tummy and keep the torso straight. Keep your knees slightly bent. Raise your arms sideways, palms down, up to shoulder level. Lower arms to sides again and raise arms upwards in front of you, again with palms down, up to shoulder level. Lower to complete movement. Continue in a side-front-side-front motion.

## ALL FOURS SUPERMAN
## WITH ALTERNATING ARMS

Start on the floor on your hands and knees. While holding that position, raise your right arm and left leg off of the ground. Keep the tummy tucked and the back straight. Return to the starting position and repeat with the other arm and leg. Hold each lift for 1-2 seconds. Reposition and repeat according to the required repetitions/time.

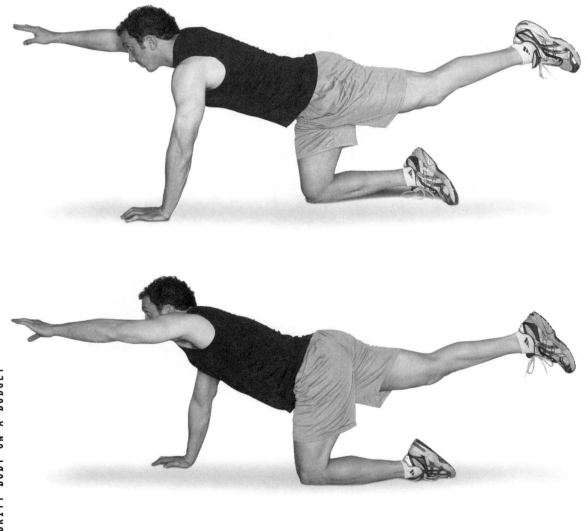

## 360-DEGREE LUNGE WITH DUMBBELLS

Start by standing with your feet shoulder width apart and holding a dumbbell in each hand. Step forward with one foot so the forward knee is directly over the toes and at a 90-degree angle. Your back knee should come close to touching the ground (6 inches away) and your front leg should be bent to about 90 degrees at the knee. Maintain your upright posture throughout the movement. Push back to the starting position as you slightly swivel your entire body on the balls of the rear leg and continue with the same leg. Keep turning in the same direction until you have completed a full circle. Repeat on the opposite leg in the opposite direction for the same number of repetitions.

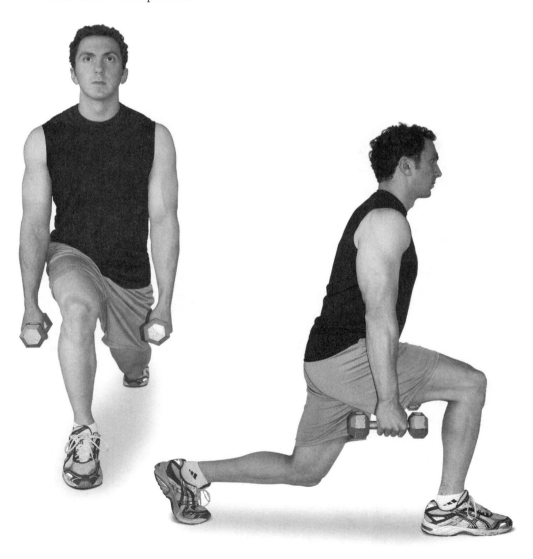

## WALL SIT

With your back against a wall and your feet about 2 feet away from the wall, slide down until your knees are at a 90-degree angle. Make sure that your knees don't extend beyond your toes. Hold the position for 30-60 seconds (longer if you can), then return to an upright position to complete this exercise.

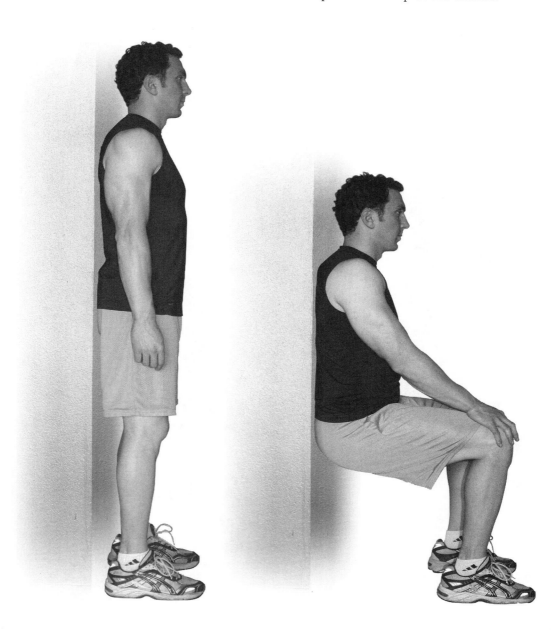

## CURL TO PRESS

Start by standing with your feet shoulder width apart
and holding a dumbbell in each hand. Keep knees
slightly bent and the back straight. With palms turned
inward curl dumbbells up to shoulders. As you begin
to extend your arms above your head, twist both wrists
so palms now face forward. Lower weights in the same
order as you raised them and continue this in the same
smooth motion.

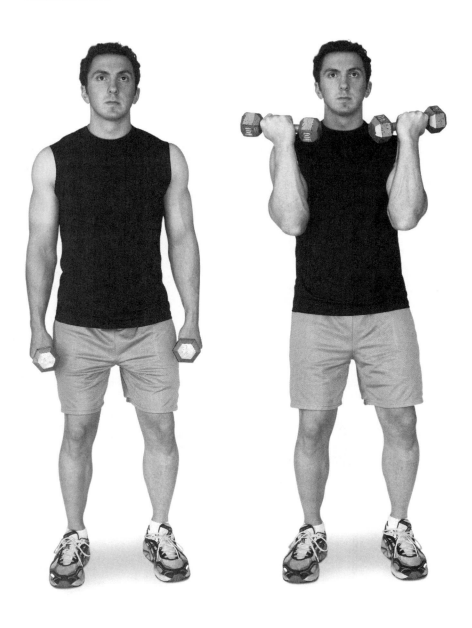

## THE PLANK

Lie face down on a mat resting on the forearms, palms flat on the floor. Push off the floor, raising up onto the balls of your feet and resting on the elbows. Tilt your pelvis and contract your abdominal muscles by drawing your navel inward toward your spine and brace it there. Keep your back straight (don't collapse in the middle) in a straight line from head to heels. Hold this position for set amount of time/repetitions.

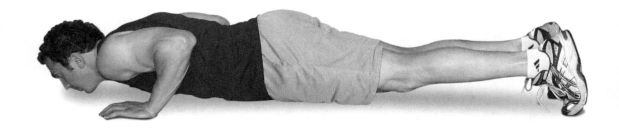

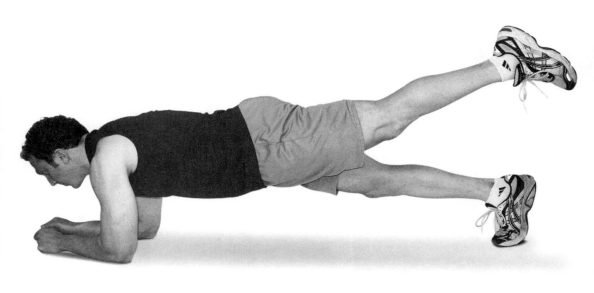

## HIGH KNEES SPRINTS

Sprinting on the spot with high knee lift, pick your knees up to waist height and pump your arms. Speed of movements and/or height of knees determine intensity. Continue to the end.

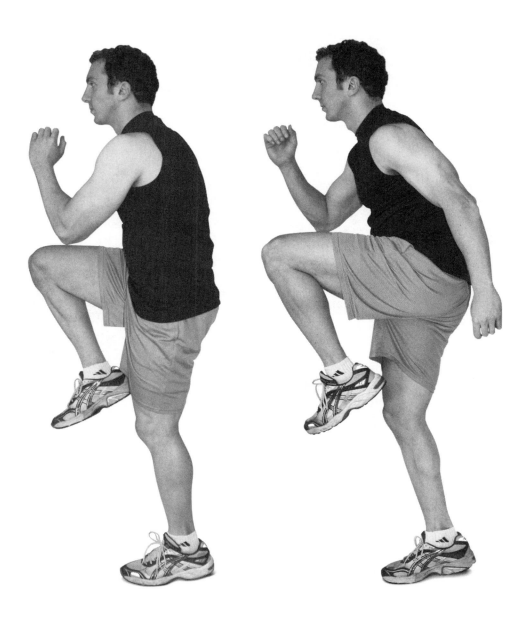

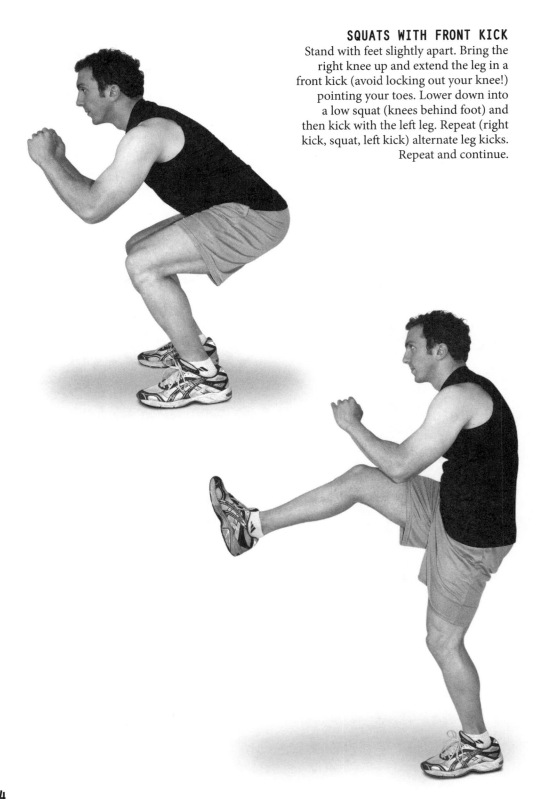

## SQUATS WITH FRONT KICK
Stand with feet slightly apart. Bring the right knee up and extend the leg in a front kick (avoid locking out your knee!) pointing your toes. Lower down into a low squat (knees behind foot) and then kick with the left leg. Repeat (right kick, squat, left kick) alternate leg kicks. Repeat and continue.

## DUMBBELL OVERHEAD SWINGS

Hold a dumbbell in each hand at your sides. Keep
your knees and elbows slightly bent and the torso
tilting slightly forward. Start the movement by
raising the dumbbells upward over your head as you
keep your palms facing inward. Gradually lower
weights to the starting position and repeat.

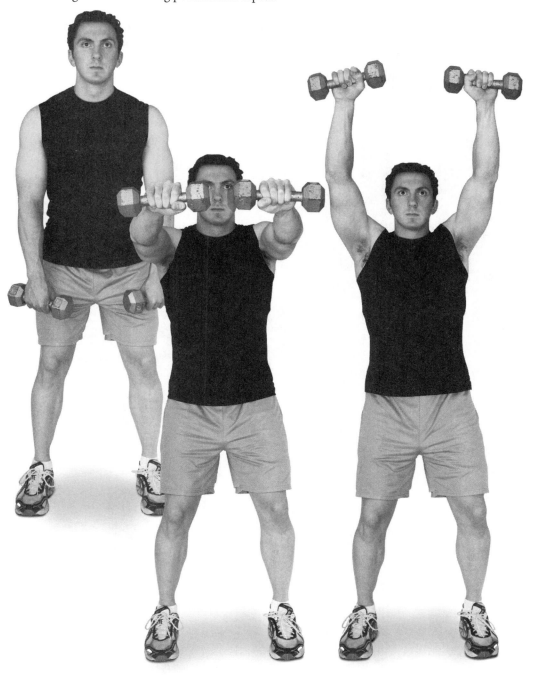

## COMPASS JUMPS

Imagine you are standing in the center of a compass—north is to your front. Hop with both legs forward to the north position and then hop back to the center, hop to the right and then back to the center, hop backwards and back to the center, and finally hop to the left and back to the center. Repeat this action rhythmically and continuously without stopping for the allotted time/repetitions.

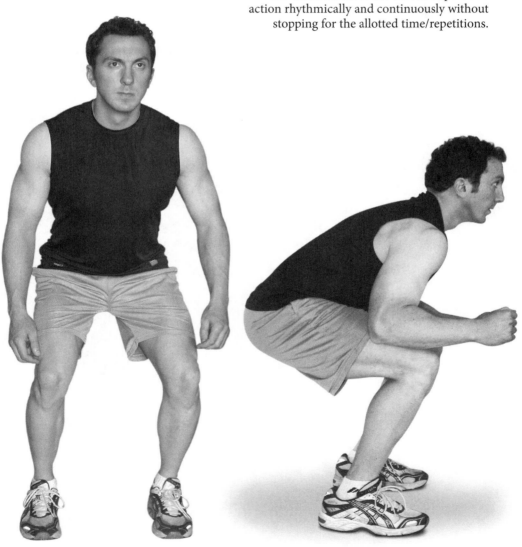

## DIAGONAL REACHES

Lie on your back and bend both knees, with your feet together and flat on the floor. Place your free hand on your opposite thigh. Keep a gap between chin and chest. Contract the abs and curl your shoulder blades off the floor and slide your hand up your thigh with slight twist to the side where your hand is placed. Lower and repeat.

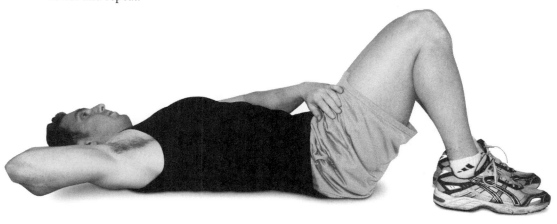

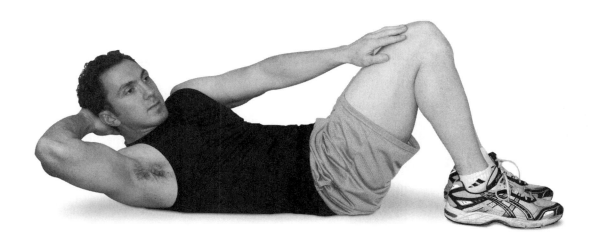

# SPECIALIST EXERCISER PROGRAM

Begin with 3 circuits and 12 repetitions for each exercise. Perform this routine 3 times a week on non-consecutive days. Consult the chart below for a weekly progress plan. The numbers in the chart suggest the amount of circuits followed by the amount of repetitions you should perform. After completing the sixth week of this program, variety will be important in order to continually stimulate the body into further improvement. Attempt one or more of the following variations for the next four weeks:

1. Add an additional repetition to each exercise within each circuit.

2. Add an additional circuit.

3. Change the exercise order in each circuit.

4. Use timed circuits. For example, consider performing each exercise for one minute straight in the first circuit, 45 seconds in the second circuit, and perhaps 30 seconds in the third circuit.

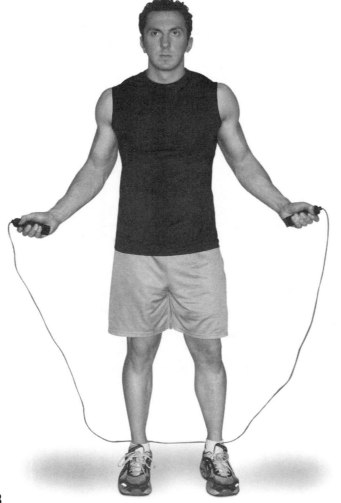

|  | Circuit x Reps |
|---|---|
| Week 1 | 3 x 12 |
| Week 2 | 3 x 14 |
| Week 3 | 3 x 16 |
| Week 4 | 3 x 18 |
| Week 5 | 3 x 20 |
| Week 6 | 3 x 22 |

## JUMPING ROPE/ SKIPPING (WITH OR WITHOUT A ROPE)

There are various types of skipping. Use variations and be creative with your movements. Try two feet off the ground, alternate feet, hop on one leg for 5 counts then swap, and so on. Jump for 30 seconds to 1 minute. Jump on one foot for half the time and switch legs for the remainder, jumping only an inch or so off the floor.

## PLYOMETRIC PUSH-UPS

Same as a regular push-up except as you extend
your arms push up explosively so your hands leave
the ground. Then allow your elbows to bend slightly
to absorb the shock as you land. Lower and repeat.
A variation of this exercise is to quickly clap your
hands as they are in the air. Keep your stomach
muscles braced and your back straight.

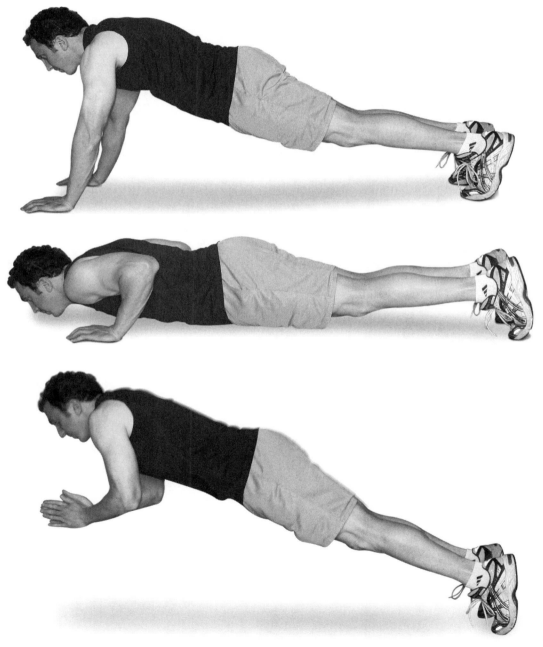

## TUCK JUMP

Standing on the spot, explosively jump up so both legs leave the ground simultaneously and tuck both knees in toward your chest. Land softly onto the balls of your feet first, then press down your heels to absorb the impact as you land with both feet at the same time. Repeat rhythmically and continuously for the allotted time/repetitions.

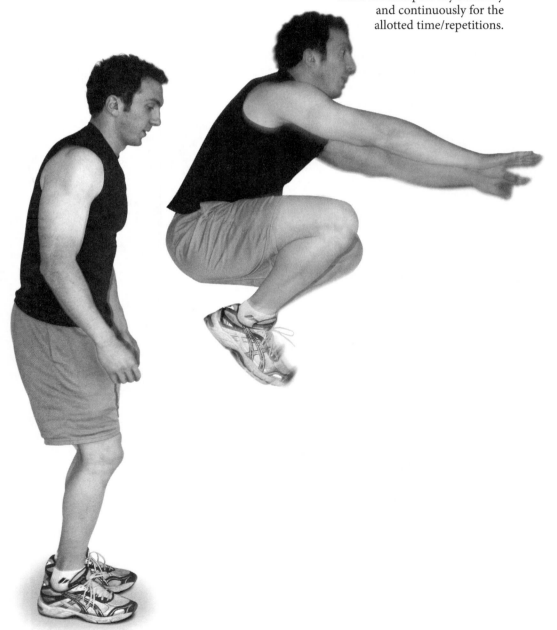

## LONG ARM CRUNCHES

Lie on your back and extend the arms straight out behind the head with hands clasped, keeping upper arms next to the ears. Contract the abs and lift the shoulder blades off the floor. Keep the arms straight and cradle the head with your arms to avoid neck strain. Lower and repeat for the allotted time/repetitions.

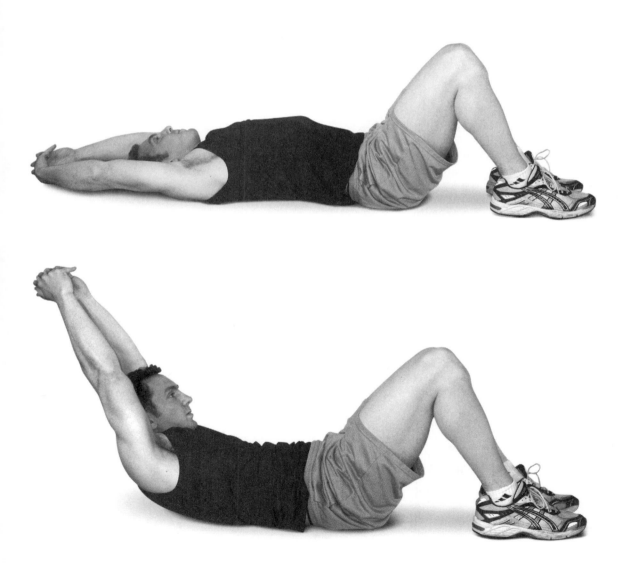

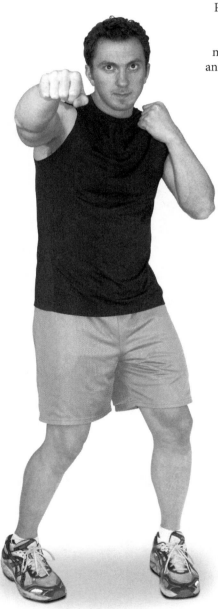

## SHADOW BOXING

Assume a boxing position and go for a little shadow boxing. Focus on controlled movements (not flailing punches), stay light on the balls of your feet and keep your knees bent. Practice jabs, power punches, hooks, and upper cuts. Hold a pair of very light weights or bottles of water for more resistance. Repeat rhythmically and continuously for the allotted time.

## CHAIR DIPS

Place two chairs facing each other (or a bed and a chair or bench, etc.) about 3 feet apart. Sit on one chair with your hands palm down and gripping the edge of the chair. Place your heels on the edge of the other chair and hold yourself up using your upper arms. Slide forward just far enough that your buttocks clears the edge of the chair and lower yourself so your elbows are at 90 degrees. Extend up again to return to start position. Lower and repeat for the allotted time/repetitions.

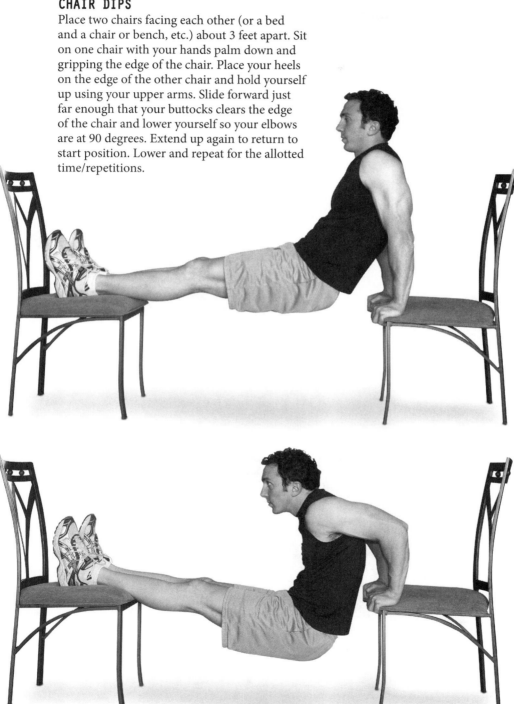

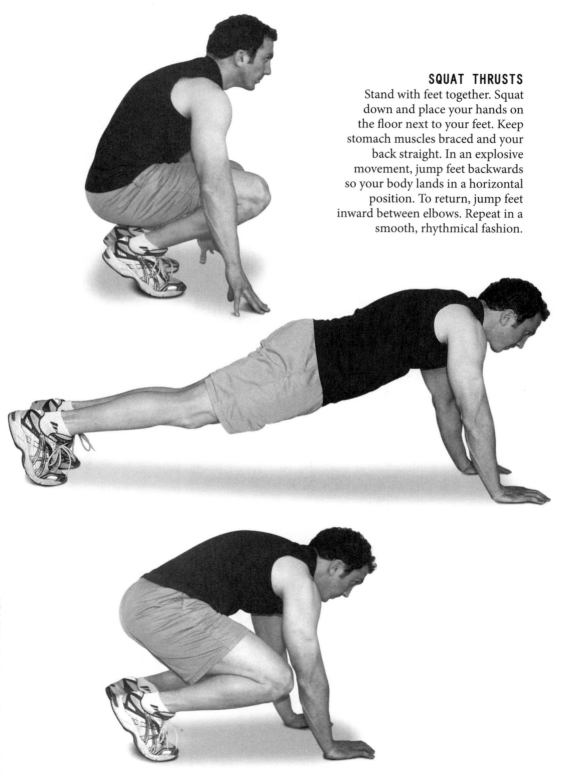

## SQUAT THRUSTS

Stand with feet together. Squat down and place your hands on the floor next to your feet. Keep stomach muscles braced and your back straight. In an explosive movement, jump feet backwards so your body lands in a horizontal position. To return, jump feet inward between elbows. Repeat in a smooth, rhythmical fashion.

## VERTICAL REVERSE CURL

Lie face up on the floor and extend the legs straight up with ankles crossed, arms by your sides. Contract your abs to lift the hips off the floor by pushing upward with your legs. Keep the legs in a fixed position and imagine bringing your belly button toward your spine at the top of the movement. Lower and repeat for the designated repetitions/time.

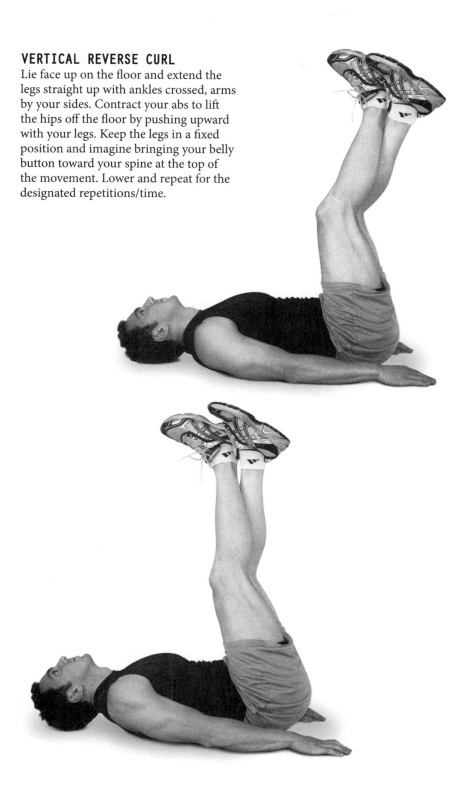

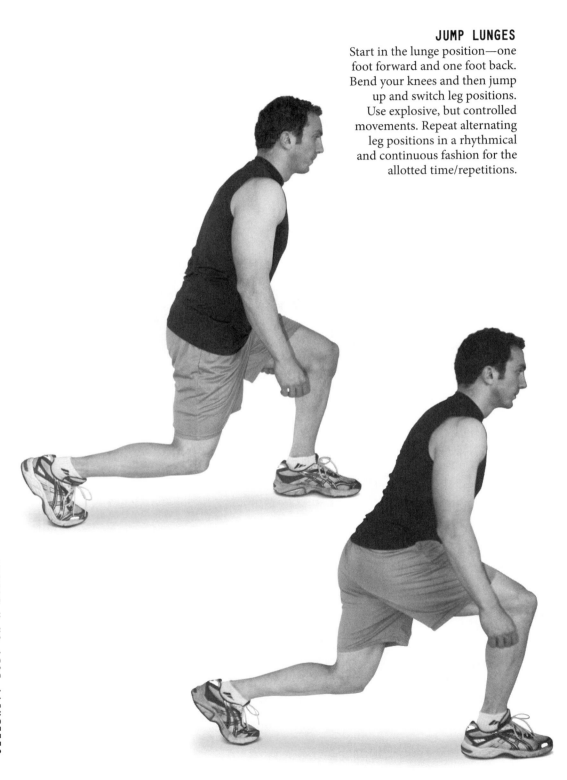

## JUMP LUNGES

Start in the lunge position—one foot forward and one foot back. Bend your knees and then jump up and switch leg positions. Use explosive, but controlled movements. Repeat alternating leg positions in a rhythmical and continuous fashion for the allotted time/repetitions.

## ALTERNATE ARM CURLS

Hold a dumbbell, water bottle, or strength band in each hand. Stand with legs hip width apart and knees slightly soft. Brace your abs and keep your back straight. Place your elbows at your sides. With palms facing upward, curl one arm up to your shoulders. Extend arm again to lower to starting position, as you curl other arm. Carry on in this alternating fashion for selected length of time.

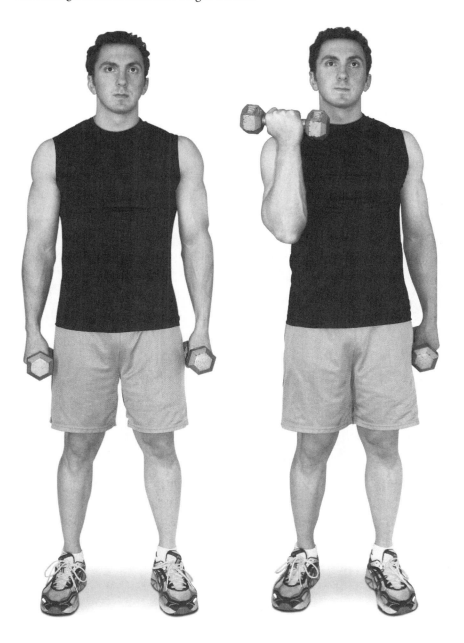

## SCISSOR STEP-UPS

Use a step or bench that is approximately mid-shin to knee height. Put your left foot on the step, with your right foot on the floor and your arms at your sides. Then push down with your left leg and drive your body upward rapidly, switching support (hopping) from left foot to right foot as your body reaches its maximal vertical height. With your right foot supporting your body, lower the left foot to the floor rapidly but under control. Repeat this action continuously, back and forth from foot to foot, without pausing at the top or bottom positions.

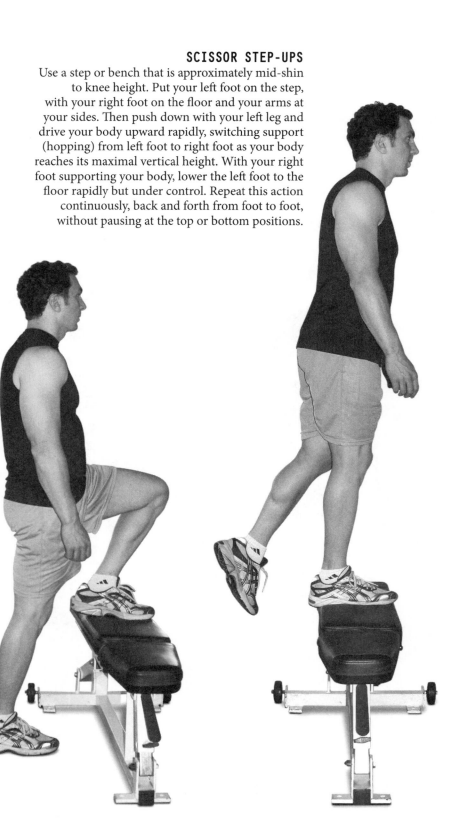

## PLANK WITH LEG EXTENSION

In the all-fours position on your mat, rest on the forearms with palms flat on the floor. Push off the floor, raising up onto balls of feet and resting on the elbows. Tilt your pelvis and contract your abdominal muscles by drawing your navel inward toward your spine and brace it there. Keep your back straight (don't collapse in the middle) in a straight line from head to heels. Slowly lift one leg while keeping hips and shoulders square. Switch legs, holding this position for the indicated number of seconds on each side.

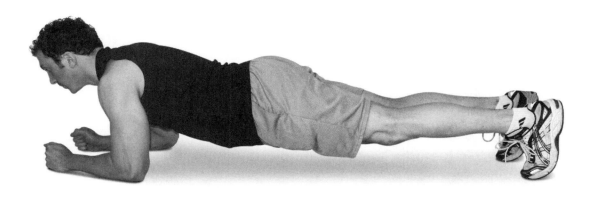

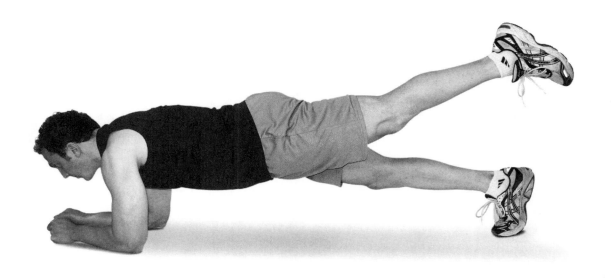

## SQUAT JUMPS

Stand with feet shoulder width apart, torso tilted forward slightly, and back straight. Arms should be in the "ready" position with elbows bent at approximately right angles. Bend legs so thighs are parallel to ground. Explode vertically and drive arms up.

Land softly onto the balls of your feet first, then press down your heels to absorb the impact as you land with both feet at the same time. Repeat rhythmically and continuously.

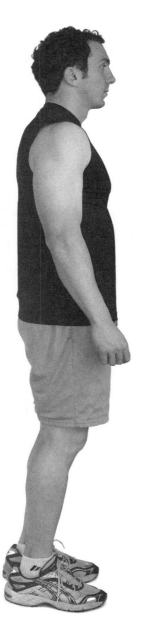

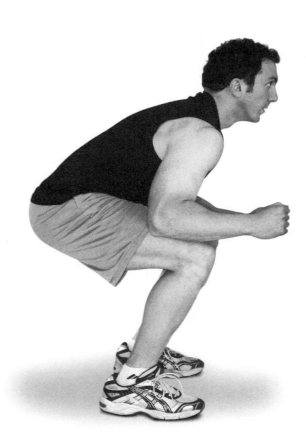

## PUSH-UP SIDE PLANK COMBO

In push-up position (on hands and balls of feet), perform one push-up. As you come up, shift weight to your left arm and twist to the side while bringing the right arm up toward the ceiling in a side plank. Keep abdominal muscles braced and the spine and back straight. Lower the arm back to the floor for another push-up and then twist to the other side. Repeat.

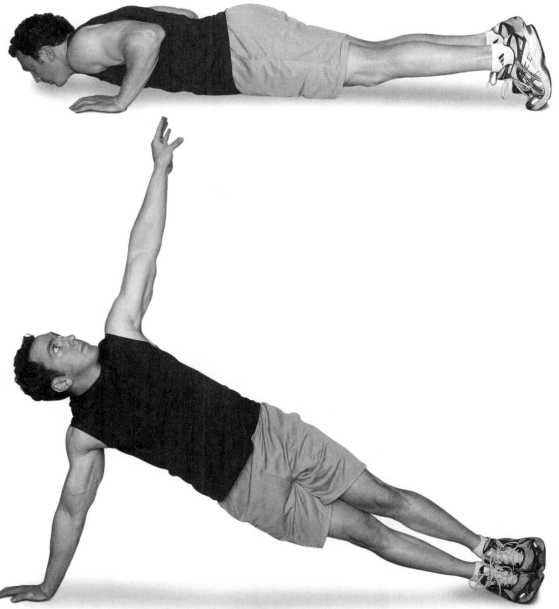

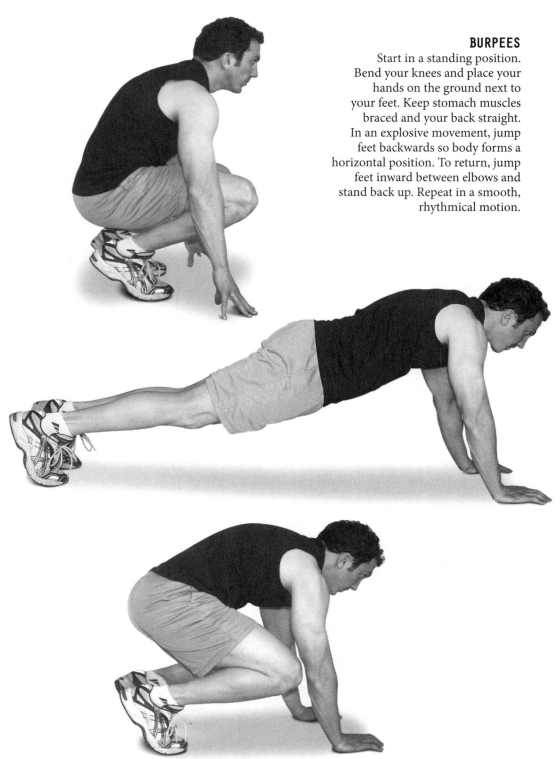

## BURPEES

Start in a standing position. Bend your knees and place your hands on the ground next to your feet. Keep stomach muscles braced and your back straight. In an explosive movement, jump feet backwards so body forms a horizontal position. To return, jump feet inward between elbows and stand back up. Repeat in a smooth, rhythmical motion.

## V-UPS

Lie back onto floor with knees bent and hands extended toward ceiling. Head should be in a neutral position with a space between chin and chest. Leading with the chin and chest toward the ceiling, contract the abdominal muscles and raise your shoulders off the floor. At the same time, raise your legs up toward the ceiling and attempt to touch your hands to your feet. Return to starting position and repeat.

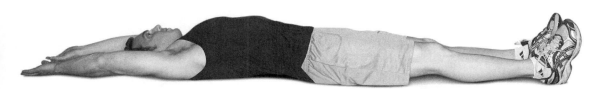

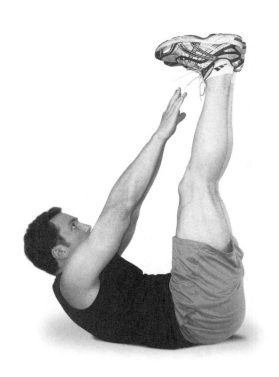

### SQUAT TO PRESSES

Holding a relatively light dumbbell in each hand by your side, stand with feet hip width apart. Squat down until your knees are bent just above 90 degrees. As you extend your legs, push the dumbbells overhead and extend your arms fully. Lower the weights as you squat down again. Repeat and continue.

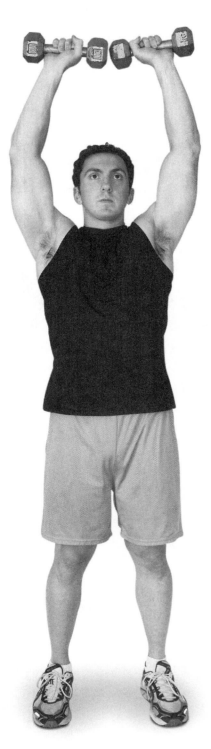

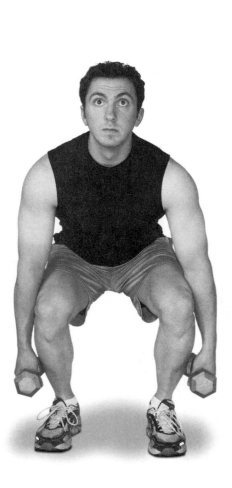

## ALTERNATING SPLIT SQUAT

Stand with feet hip width apart. Step back with your left leg approximately 2 feet standing on the ball of your back foot. Feet should be positioned at a staggered stance with the head and back erect and straight in a neutral position. Place your hands on your waist. Lower your body by bending at the right hip and knee until your thigh is parallel to the floor then immediately explode vertically. Switch feet in the air so that the back foot lands forward and vice versa. Repeat in a smooth, rhythmical motion.

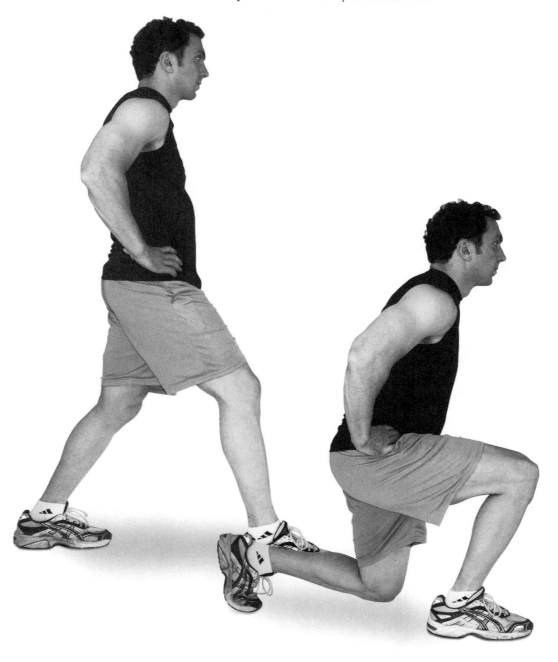

# CHAPTER
## *Six:*
## EAT IT TO BEAT IT

CHAPTER SIX:

# EAT IT TO *beat* IT

Healthy eating is the last thing on many people's minds when purse strings are tight. As we look to save cash, good quality and nutritious produce are often swapped in favor of cheaper canned goods and processed foods. It's easy to lose sight of your body, and even if you wish to lose those extra pounds, you may feel bound by your financial limitations. But, with thought and planning, it is possible to eat well without making a large dent in your weekly food budget.

Food prices have been soaring recently. Cash-strapped families are being forced to change the way they shop and cook in a bid to make family meals go further. Perhaps your healthy shopping list is starting to seem expensive, especially when you see tempting promotional offers on cookies, potato chips, and multi-packs of sweets. But you can—with the help of a few tips and tricks—save money and still eat well.

People seem to have the misconception that cutting back on food expenses means giving up healthy foods. However, it doesn't necessarily have to be more expensive to eat healthier!

There can be many positive outcomes from tough financial times; a tighter budget actually can guide us to a healthier diet. It's an interesting fact that people were better fed during, and just after, World War II, when there wasn't much money or food around. People didn't eat so much processed food and stuck to food that was fairly fresh.

## CHANGE THE WAY YOU BUY FOOD AND COOK

Everyone has to eat, and food makes up a significant proportion of every family's expenses. But there are ways to spend less, yet still eat well. All it takes is some advance planning. This book understands the temptations of purchasing unhealthy food when trying to maintain a financial budget. Take a closer look at this book's ideas and give them a try.

# HOW TO BE A HEALTHY FOOD SAVVY SHOPPER

1. **BE PREPARED.** If you're going to be out running errands or shopping with your family, bring some healthy snacks and drinks with you. That way, if hunger pangs strike, you won't be tempted to stop at a fast food restaurant or buy snacks from a vending machine—something that can hurt your wallet and your waistline. Whether you make snacks at home or buy them from the grocery store, it's less expensive than buying them in an overpriced café or restaurant.

2. **PLAN YOUR MEALS AND ONLY BUY WHAT YOU NEED.** If you often end up discarding precious food because it's gone bad before you've had a chance to use it, try setting aside some time each week to write a list of meals for the week ahead. Produce a detailed shopping list from that plan, and aim to stick to it when you get to the supermarket. Remember, supermarkets want you to impulse buy. That's how they make money. But that is also how it is easy to end up spending far more than you intended. Also, it's usually cheaper to buy larger quantities, so by organizing your main meals in advance, you'll be using some of the same fresh ingredients two or three times during the week.

3. **TAKE ADVANTAGE OF SHOPPING INCENTIVES.** If your store offers a frequent shopper program, usually in the form of a swipe card, definitely sign up to receive advanced notice of special offers and other money-saving information. You should also keep an eye on newspapers and advertising flyers for special offers and money-off coupons, particularly on costly items such as meats, fruit, and vegetables. With money-off coupons, it's wise to proceed with caution! Be sure you use coupons only for products you would normally buy anyway. Watch for sales on those items in addition to your coupons and multiply your savings. Coupons can be a Catch-22 because often times they apply to foods that are more expensive in the first place. Used wisely, however, coupons can also be a great cost saver.

4. **CREATE YOUR OWN STORE PRICE BOOK.** This neat and simple system will help you track store prices so that when you see an item on sale, you'll immediately know whether it's a good deal or not. You'll want to record the date, store, item, size, price, and sale price. Admittedly, however, this system isn't for everyone, as it can be time consuming, but you may find it a useful practice. Do some price comparisons among grocery stores. Often you can do this right online, saving you the need to drive around to all the different stores.

5. **BUY IN BULK. IF YOU CAN AFFORD IT, BUY IN BULK.** Large quantities are cheaper, and some discount grocery stores will often give good deals for those who buy by the box. However, buying twice your usual amount of snack foods because they're on sale doesn't always mean they'll last twice as long in the cupboard. The more we buy, the faster we tend to go through it. So don't stock up on those super-sized packets of potato chips just because they're a great deal this week. Instead, look for buy-one-get-one-free deals on longer shelf life cupboard staples such as dried pasta, canned tuna, canned vegetables, breads, and anything else that will keep well or which you can freeze. Remember, be sensible by buying in bulk, but buy the right foods.

6. **AVOID PREPACKAGED FOODS,** such as ready meals, pre-cut vegetables, or diced meats—they tend to be much more expensive. Ready-to-cook meats are also more expensive, for example, marinated boneless chicken or seasoned roasts. A cheaper option is to purchase plain meat and prepare it yourself at home.

7. **VARY WHERE YOU SHOP.** Visit your local ethnic food store or local fresh food market for a variety of different foods not available at mainstream stores. It can be a great way to save money, particularly if you buy in bulk.

8. **CHOOSE A CHEAPER SUPERMARKET.** Don't dismiss the idea of switching to a cheaper store for part of your weekly shopping trip. For most items, such as canned goods and paper products, the quality is unlikely to vary much since most supermarkets carry many the same national brands. The big difference may come in fresh foods and private store brands. You can realize a significant saving by buying some of your groceries at a less expensive store.

9. **BUY LOCAL PRODUCE AND FRUITS AND VEGETABLES THAT ARE IN SEASON.** Local, seasonal produce is usually cheaper than foods that have to be imported. Fresher fruit and vegetables taste better. Not only is it better for your wallet and taste buds, but it's better for the environment. Your food won't have clocked hundreds or even thousands of road miles on its way to your dinner table.

10. **EXPERIMENT WITH STORE BRANDS;** most of the time the only difference is in the price, not the quality of the food. If buying processed goods, supermarkets' own brands are significantly cheaper than national brands and often are made by the same manufacturer.

11. **GO FROZEN.** Another option is to go for frozen produce, which prevents wastage and is more cost effective. Because much of your food budget is likely to be spent on protein, it's smart to have a freezer. That way you can stock up at sales of lean ground beef, turkey, chuck roast, and other healthy meats that will stay fresh in the freezer for six to nine months. Frozen vegetables are usually cheaper than anything that can be found in the produce and canned sections of the store. Cruise down the frozen food aisles, and you'll find big bags of vegetables at bargain prices.

12. **SHOP WHEN PRODUCTS ARE REDUCED.** When possible, shop late in the day, when supermarkets discount products that will not keep. Most stores will cut prices on their perishable foodstuffs near the end of the day. Check the "use by" date. Go shopping an hour or two before the store closes. You'll always be able to pick up some great bargains. Bread, fruit, and vegetables as well as chilled foods are the best products to look for. If you know you'll use the food by the expiration date, great! Go for it! But if you're not sure, you could wind up wasting that food, which wastes your funds. If you find a good deal on a soon-to-expire product, it's worthwhile to purchase it if it's a food that can be frozen, as this will keep it fresh for some time. You can make significant savings that way.

13. **AVOID THE "DIET" PRODUCTS.** Not to be confused with "light" versions of foods, although low-fat products are often more expensive than their regular equivalents. "Diet" products are those overpriced shakes, meal replacement bars, energy gels, and other weird and wonderful potions that bear little relation to actual food. These are all cost inflated and often of questionable nutritional value.

14. **SAY NO TO RIP-OFF BOTTLED WATER.** One of the biggest savings can come from buying a water jug with a filter or by installing a filter to your tap instead of lugging home bottled water. You'll also be doing a good deed for the environment—no more plastic bottles! Immense savings can be made if you consider the cost of how much water you consume over the week. The cost of a jug with a filter will easily be recovered within just a few weeks. The payback time on a tap-fitted filter will be longer due to the cost of installation and a more sophisticated filter, but still well worth it.

15. **EDUCATE YOURSELF.** Study the basic nutrition information on food labels to help you make the most nutritious choices for you and your family. Use the nutrition facts label to focus on the facts that are most important to you such as the fat, sugar, or sodium content. Nutritional labels also make it easier for you to compare similar products.

16. **SHOP ONLINE.** Take advantage of supermarkets that offer online shopping. Even though many charge for the service (a delivery fee usually), you'll be surprised how much you could save by avoiding the temptation to fill your cart with impulse purchases. You'll also save time and a little on fuel and wear and tear on your car if your supermarket happens to be miles away.

17. **USE A CASH BACK OR REWARDS CREDIT CARD.** If you regularly pay your credit card bill in full at the end of the month, then a cash back credit card could benefit you. For every dollar you spend on one of these cards, you receive a percentage back. Cash back bonuses are usually paid annually, so you could treat yourself to a little something extra with your rebate.

18. **FINALLY, MY FAVORITE TIP IS TO EAT BEFORE YOU SHOP.** The old, but tried and tested tip—never shop on an empty stomach—is true! If you shop hungry, you'll be more likely to impulsively buy, rather than sticking to what you actually need. So, if you're feeling peckish when you shop, you'll pile the cart higher. So make sure you grab a healthy snack and a glass of water to fill yourself up before filling your shopping cart.

## WEED IT AND REAP

In tough times, it's wise to make sure the only crunch you feel is the bite of your homegrown carrots. You could save money, get fit, enrich your social life, do your bit for the environment, and be super-trendy all at once with your own garden.

Start a gardening plot in your backyard. A corner of the garden or a container garden on your patio can be used for salad leaves, most of which require little care. Potatoes, carrots, and cabbages are also easy to grow. Asparagus is a lot of work, but the rewards are worthwhile—and you save a substantial amount of money.

If you're a lover of fresh herbs, you could try growing your favorite herbs in small pots by the kitchen window and take a snip whenever you need a particular herb to liven up dish. You really can enjoy homegrown fruits and vegetables all season long. The big bonus is you'll know exactly what has been added in the process.

# TIPS FOR TRIMMING BACK YOUR RESTAURANT BILL

Everyone wants to enjoy a meal out every once in a while. Eating out with family and friends is an expensive luxury in life most of us enjoy, no matter how budget-minded we are. It is a pleasurable way to get out of the house and let someone else do the cooking. It is also an easy activity to cut out when you're trying to juggle your finances. But you don't have to become a hermit and miss out entirely on your favorite chef's specialties.

1.  **GIVE THE APPETIZERS A TRY.** If your eyes are not bigger than your belly, try out the appetizers before tucking into the main course menu. You can often order an exquisite appetizer and a mixed salad with water and lemon for well under the cost of a main course. To really fill you up, ask for fresh bread to accompany your meal. If you're still tempted by a main course in addition to your appetizer, share it with someone, which most restaurants allow (although some add a small plate charge) to save on cost.

2.  **STARVE THAT SWEET TOOTH OF YOURS.** Try to avoid ordering dessert. Not only are the majority of restaurant desserts calorie laden, the cost often exceeds that of the appetizer and can sometimes cost as much as a main course. If you simply cannot resist having a dessert, order one dessert, accompanied by extra forks, and share it with your dining companions.

3.  **AVOID PEAK TIME DINING.** If you have been itching to try an expensive restaurant in your area, go for a late lunch and avoid the higher dinner prices. Take advantage of early bird specials at restaurants— usually offered between 4:00 p.m. to 6:00 p.m. Until recently, restaurants served the same menu items for less money during early bird hours, but now they're likely to serve smaller portions for less money. Of course, trimming portions translates into fewer calories, fewer extra pounds on the scale, and fewer dollars out of your dining out budget. Restaurants' tendency to super-size has led us to expect larger portions than we need. Lunchtime menus are usually a lot cheaper, and you're less likely to spend as much on extras such as wine. And before you leave the house, check online to see if you can track down some printable restaurant discount vouchers or voucher codes that can be used in conjunction with the final bill.

4. **GO DUTCH.** Take along a friend when possible and take advantage of the buy-one-get-one-free or two-for-the-price-of-one deals often advertised in newspapers or Web sites. Simply total the bill (including the tip) and divide it into however many diners are present. You will all save money.

5. **SEEK OUT KID'S NIGHT DEALS.** Most family restaurants offer specials such as free meals for kids when adults order a meal, discounts on kids' meals, freebies such as a free dessert with a meal, and other cost-cutting deals. Restaurants often run kids' specials during the week on slow evenings such as Tuesdays and Wednesdays. Call and find out if your favorite family restaurant offers this type of promotion.

6. **THINK BEFORE YOU DRINK.** One of the biggest income streams for all restaurants is the drinks list. Alcohol, soft drinks, tea, and coffee add significantly to your bill. Substitute bottled water or a glass of tap water with a slice of lemon and/or wait until you are home to have your after-dinner coffee. By ordering wine with dinner, you can watch your savings dwindle away before your very eyes. The cost to you for just one glass of house wine is the equivalent to what the restaurant pays for the entire bottle. The restaurant easily creams off 400 percent to 500 percent profit. So think of what you're paying for when you buy by the glass!

7. **GO FETCH THE DOGGIE BAG.** If you're eyes were bigger than your appetite, don't struggle to finish your meal. Ask for a doggie bag. Take the leftovers home and have them for lunch the next day. It is a great way to economize—turning one large meal into two meals.

8. **SIGN UP AND BE REWARDED.** Many popular restaurants offer special savings and reward programs, which you can receive if you subscribe to their Web site newsletter (the same applies to some supermarket promotions). Many advertise that by joining their online programs, you will receive from time to time special promotions and coupons through e-mail. Simply print out the vouchers and take them along for a great dining experience minus the mega-bucks! Massive savings can be achieved through this measure.

Remember, you work hard, so why not enjoy an evening out once in a while? Try using some of the tips in this chapter before cutting dining out—out of your budget!

# HEY, GOOD LOOKING, WHAT YA GOT COOKING!

If you're trying to eat healthy, the question is where to cut back while getting the most nutritious food possible. There's no reason to stop eating healthy, nutritious, tasty food during hard economic times. In fact, now is a great time to experiment with various types of food. So what are you waiting for? Use these *Celebrity Body on a Budget* tips to get you in the mood.

1. **COUNT ALL THE COSTS.** You want a trimmer body, without a slimmer wallet. But when you're cutting calories, it's not always easy to cut costs. If you're not careful, fresh salads, juicy fruits, and lean meats can add up to far more than the value meal at McDonald's or that economy-size box of macaroni and cheese. What's a cost-conscious dieter to do? The first thing to keep in mind is this: When you count the costs of a healthier diet, don't forget to tally the costs of being overweight.

2. **CONSIDER HOW MUCH NUTRITION YOU'RE GETTING FOR YOUR MONEY.** Prepackaged, boxed, canned, and frozen foods often contain more fat, calories, sodium, and sugar and can be expensive compared to preparing your own meals from scratch. In addition, they can be lacking in vital nutrients such as vitamins and minerals.

3. **GO BACK TO THE BASICS.** Cook from basic ingredients. Cooking from scratch rather than using canned items and packets is far cheaper— and healthier. And often it doesn't take as long as you think. If you're pressured for time, you can cook in the microwave or cook a week's worth of meals and freeze them in individual portions.

4. **DON'T LEAVE OUT LEFTOVERS.** It's easy to use up leftovers by turning them into pies, soups, and stews. Leftovers can be separated into small portions that are dated and frozen. Don't freeze and then thaw a large portion of food (more than you'll eat in a serving) because you'll end up wasting most of it. Dry cheese can be grated and added to soups rather than thrown away, and stale bread makes excellent breadcrumbs or croutons.

5. **CONSIDER THE MATTER OF TIME.** Time is a factor in the popularity of bagged salads, grated cheese, cut-up apples and veggies, and similar convenience items. If you want to be frugal, wash your own greens, grate your own cheese, and slice your own apples and vegetables. The mark up on the prepared versions is huge.

6. **DON'T COMPROMISE ON TASTE.** Eating drab, dull food isn't the way to go. Eating on a budget doesn't have to mean eating nothing but white refined pasta or regular ground meat. Resist fatty foods! They may be cheap, but the hidden costs can add up fast. Being unhealthy and overweight won't save you any money.

7. **GET THE "FILL" OF IT.** Carbohydrates are "fill-you-up" food. They're cheap, and they give you energy. However, make sure you skip the refined "white" carbohydrates; instead, look for the browns. Choose unrefined rye, whole wheat, spelt flour, and brown rice.

8. **GET BY WITH A LITTLE HELP FROM YOUR FRIENDS.** Ask friends and family to help you out with the cooking. Get them to share ideas with you. Variety is important, and with more than one cook in the household, you won't get into a rut. Cooking can be a form of entertainment for everyone. Talk to your spouse, your roommates, your friends, or your children about what they'd like to eat and how they can make it on a budget.

9. **DISCOVER NEW (AND OLD) RECIPES.** Chances are your grandmother's family recipes were economical. Perhaps you remember her talking about some old classic and favorite dishes. Phone or e-mail your older relatives and ask if they have any good recipes to share from the past. Those meals from past times may have tasted good, but they probably weren't all healthy. Today there's more information available than ever before about healthy cooking in general, vegetarianism, and veganism. Go out and find it! Do a few Internet searches or check out a book full of great new recipes at the library.

10. **GET SAUCY.** Slash the fat grams in your cakes, muffins, and other baked items by replacing the oil in recipes with an equal amount of no-sugar-added apple sauce. It won't change the taste of your recipe, but it will change the healthfulness of it.

11. **DON'T BE AN EGGHEAD.** Reduce your cholesterol consumption by substituting the eggs in baked goods with a tablespoon of soy flour. You can pick up a bag for a small sum of money, and it will last you for quite a long time.

12. **HALT THE SALT.** Sodium lurks in lots of foods, and it's just not something that your body needs in large quantities. Limit your consumption by purchasing no-salt-added or low-sodium versions of canned foods. This switch won't cost you a penny, so it's probably the simplest switch of all.

13. **DUMP THE JUNK.** Sugary soft drinks, potato chips, and cookies are a major drain on the family budget. Instead of eating this highly processed junk, try baking your own cookies and cakes or switching to water, tea, and coffee rather than the more expensive sugar-laden alternatives. A cheaper and healthier substitute to potato chips would be unbuttered popcorn.

14. **GET YOUR CREATIVE JUICES FLOWING.** You can still eat well. All it takes is imagination and a sense of adventure. Invest in spices to liven up your meals. Experiment with sauces. Prepare them in large quantities and freeze or preserve them. Make your own stock and freeze it in containers that will be ready when you want soup or stew. Curries, stews, and stir-fries are great ways to stretch meat or use leftovers.

15. **BE A MEAL STRETCHER.** You can extend your meals by adding extra vegetables and grains. For example, when cooking spaghetti Bolognese substitute half the meat for canned beans, onions, and carrots. This will save money and make the dish healthier.

16. **FREEZE FOR EASE.** Cook extra portions of curries, soups, stews, and casseroles and place them in the freezer for a later date. One-pot dishes save on preparation time, money, and dish washing— and they are the perfect option if you have a chronically busy schedule.

## TOP 12 CELEBRITY BODY ON A BUDGET *Recipes*

This book brings you the ultimate twelve easy and healthy recipes for keeping meal prices down. Here are just a few delicious and nutritious main course recipes, which will help you stay within your budget. Once you get the hang of it, you will save money on your food shopping bill and still be able to prepare delicious, exciting, and nutritious recipes for yourself, your family, and your friends. Get your pots and pans out and give them a try.

## BEEF AND CABBAGE BAKE

*Notes: Serves 4, main course, hot meal, beef, pork, vegetables, herbs*

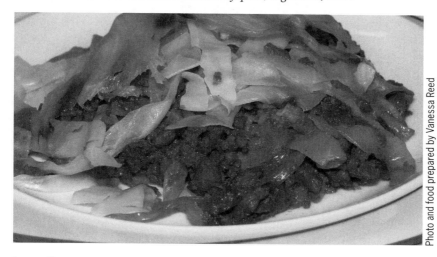

Photo and food prepared by Vanessa Reed

### Ingredients

1 medium sized white cabbage
2 onions, *chopped*
2 tablespoons olive or sunflower oil
225 g/8 oz back bacon
450 g/1 lb lean minced beef

2 beef stock cubes
150 ml/5 fl.oz water
salt and pepper
2 teaspoons dried mixed herbs
50 g/2 oz olive or sunflower spread
225 g/8 oz lean bacon

### Instructions

1. Preheat the oven to 190˚C, 375˚F, Gas mark 5.

2. Reserve 2 cabbage leaves intact then cut the remaining cabbage into quarters; remove the center core and shred. Place in a saucepan of boiling salted water with the reserved whole leaves and blanch for 2 minutes. Drain and set aside.

3. Melt the oil in a pan and gently fry the onions until transparent.
   Chop the back bacon then add to the onions and cook for 2–3 minutes.

4. Add the minced beef and brown. Crumble in the stock cubes, water, herbs, salt, and pepper and simmer for 10 minutes.

5. Melt the spread in a saucepan. Place half the cabbage in an ovenproof dish and pour the melted spread over it.

6. Spread the mince mixture over the cabbage, cover with the remaining shredded cabbage, and top with the whole cabbage leaves.

7. Arrange the lean bacon rashers over the top and bake for 45 minutes. Serve hot.

# MEATBALLS IN TOMATO SAUCE

*Notes: Serves 4, main course, hot meal, beef, vegetables, spices*

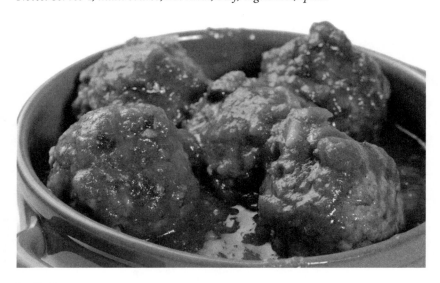

## Ingredients

150 g/5 oz crustless bread
25 g/1 oz olive or sunflower spread
1 level teaspoon dried thyme
1 onion, *grated*
1 teaspoon paprika
4 teaspoons flour

150 ml/5 fl.oz milk
a pinch of sugar
salt and pepper
450 g/1 lb lean minced beef
1 tablespoon olive oil
2210 ml/7 fl.oz beef stock
1 x 400 g/14 oz can tomatoes

## Instructions

1. Place the bread in a bowl together with the milk and leave for 30 minutes.

2. Meanwhile, melt half the spread in a pan. Sprinkle on the flour and cook for 1–2 minutes. Gradually add the stock, stirring all the time, and cook over a medium heat until thickened.

3. Add the tomatoes, sugar, and thyme to the sauce. Season well, cover, and simmer for 30 minutes.

4. Preheat the oven to 180°C, 350°F, Gas mark 4. In a bowl, mix together the minced beef, onion, soaked bread (together with the milk), paprika, salt, and pepper. Using dampened hands, roll the mixture into balls about the size of a large walnut.

5. Heat the remaining spread and oil in a large frying pan and brown the meatballs on all sides, in batches if necessary.

6. Place the meatballs in a shallow ovenproof dish, in a single layer. Pour over the tomato sauce, cover, and bake for 30 minutes. Serve hot.

# CORIANDER BEEF STEW

*Notes: Serves 4, main course, hot meal, beef, gluten, wheat and dairy free*

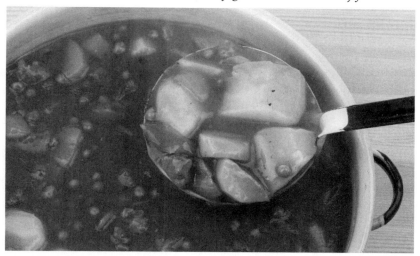

## Ingredients

3 garlic cloves, *crushed*
salt and black pepper
1 tablespoon vegetable oil
approximately 480 ml/
    16 fl. oz fresh beef stock
400 g/14 oz spinach,
    *roughly chopped*
1 large potato

2 teaspoons ground cumin
1 kg/2.2 lbs braising or stewing steak, *cubed*
1 large onion, *chopped*
1 tablespoon freshly chopped
    coriander leaves (cilantro)
180 ml/6 fl. oz water
150 g/5 oz frozen green peas
the zest of 1 lime

## Instructions

1.  In a small bowl, mix together the garlic, cumin, salt, and pepper.

2.  Place the meat in a large dish, add the garlic mixture and mix well
    with your hands. Cover and leave to marinate for at least 30 minutes.

3.  Heat the vegetable oil in a large saucepan, add the meat, and brown on all sides.

4.  Add onions and cook, stirring until soft and transparent.

5.  Add 240 ml/8 fl. oz of the stock, bring to a boil, then reduce the heat slightly
    and cook for about 45 minutes, stirring from time to time and adding
    more stock as necessary.

6.  Place the spinach and coriander in a food processor or blender
    together with 180 ml/6 fl. oz of water and process until smooth. Set aside.

7.  Peel the potato and cut into small cubes then add to the cooked meat
    together with the spinach mixture. Mix well and continue to cook for
    another 15 minutes or until the potatoes are just tender.

8.  Add the frozen peas and cook for another 5 minutes.

9.  Just before serving, stir in the lime zest. Serve hot with white rice.

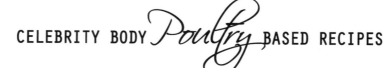

# CELEBRITY BODY *Poultry* BASED RECIPES

## CHICKEN AND BEAN STIR FRY

*Notes: Serves 4, main course, chicken, hot meal, vegetables, dairy free*

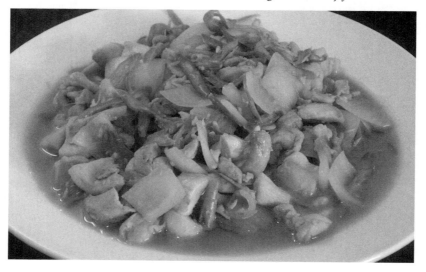

### Ingredients

2 tablespoons vegetable oil
2 garlic cloves, *crushed*
175 g/6 oz green beans,
   *thinly sliced on the diagonal*
3 tablespoons soy sauce

2 large or 4 small chicken thighs
2.5 cm/1-inch fresh root ginger, *grated*
1 onion, *cut into 2.5 cm/1-inch pieces*
100 g/4 oz small mushrooms, *halved*
120 ml/4 fl. oz hot chicken stock
juice of ½ lemon

### Instructions

1. Remove the skin and bones from the thighs and cut the flesh into 2.5 cm/1-inch pieces.

2. Heat half the oil in a large frying pan or wok until very hot then add the chicken and stir fry for 4–5 minutes until golden brown on all sides. Remove from the pan with a slotted spoon and set aside.

3. Add the remaining oil to the pan/wok and heat until hot. Add the garlic and ginger and stir fry over a medium heat for 30 seconds.

4. Increase the heat to high then add the green beans, onions, and mushrooms and stir fry for 2–3 minutes.

5. Return the cooked chicken to the pan together with the soy sauce, stock, and lemon juice. Cook for 2–3 minutes, stirring from time to time. Serve immediately.

# GINGERED CHICKEN KEBABS

*Notes: Serves 4, main course, chicken, hot meal, barbecue,*
*vegetables, dairy free, spices*

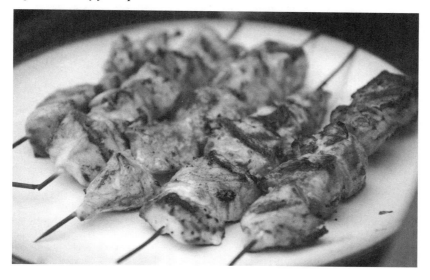

## Ingredients

450 g/1 lb boneless chicken breast or thighs
2 garlic cloves, *crushed*
5 cm/2-inch fresh ginger root, *peeled and grated*
½ teaspoon ground coriander
3 tablespoons runny honey
2 tablespoons olive oil
3 tablespoons dry sherry
2 tablespoons soy sauce
juice of ½ lime

## Instructions

1. Place all the ingredients, apart from the chicken,
   in a bowl and mix until well combined.

2. Cut the chicken into 2.5 cm/1-inch cubes and add to the marinade.
   Mix well, then cover and leave to marinate for at least 2 hours.

3. Remove the chicken from the bowl, reserving the marinade,
   and thread onto skewers.

4. Cook over medium hot coals or under a hot grill for 10–15 minutes,
   turning frequently and basting with the remaining marinade
   from time to time. Serve immediately.

# CORIANDER TURKEY BURGERS

*Notes: Serves 4, main course, turkey, hot meal, barbecue, vegetables, gluten, wheat and dairy free, spices, herbs*

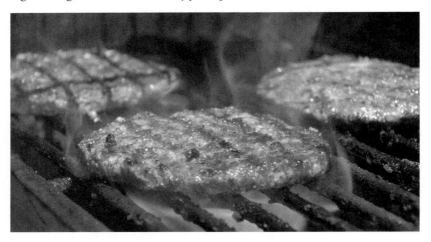

## Ingredients

450 g/1 lb turkey mince
1 small red onion, *finely chopped*
finely grated zest of 1 lime
1 heaped tablespoon freshly chopped coriander
salt and black pepper
2 tablespoons vegetable oil

## Instructions

1. Place the turkey mince, onion, lime zest, coriander, salt, and black pepper in a mixing bowl and mix well, working the mixture with your fingers.

2. Using wet hands, shape the mixture into 4 burgers about 2.5 cm/1-inch thick.

3. Heat the oil in a large frying pan, add the burgers, and fry over a medium heat for 6–8 minutes on each side or until cooked through.

Can also be cooked on the barbecue over medium/hot coals for the same length of time. Brush with oil before placing on the barbecue.

## GARLIC & MUSHROOM PASTA

*Notes: Serves 4, main course, hot meal, vegetarian, vegetables, pasta*

### Ingredients

75 g/3 oz butter
675 g/1½ lb mushrooms, *thickly sliced*
350 g/12 oz short cut pasta *(e.g., macaroni)*
juice of 1 lemon
3 garlic cloves, *chopped*
2 tablespoons fresh parsley, *chopped*
salt and black pepper

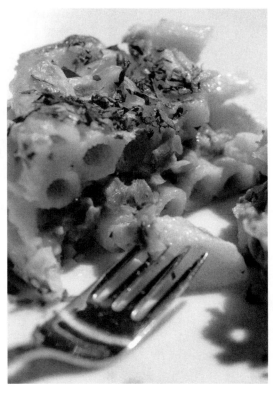

### Instructions

1. Melt the butter in a pan, add the mushrooms, cover, and cook for 10 minutes, stirring occasionally.

2. Meanwhile bring a large pan of salted water to boil, add the pasta, and cook for 10–12 minutes.

3. Add the lemon juice and garlic to the mushrooms, cover, and cook for another 5 minutes, stirring occasionally. Add the parsley, salt, and pepper and mix well.

4. To serve: drain the pasta well and toss in the sauce. Serve immediately.

# CANNELLONI WITH MUSHROOMS

*Notes: Serves 4, main course, hot meal, vegetarian, vegetables, pasta*

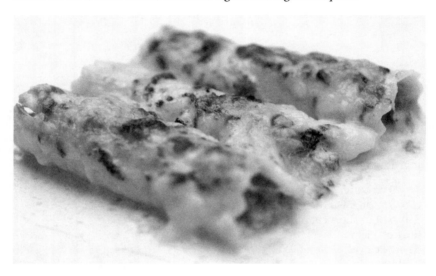

## Ingredients

8 cannelloni tubes
salt and pepper
100 g/4 oz frozen peas
50 g/2 oz butter
175 g/6 oz mushrooms, *sliced*
1 tablespoon freshly chopped basil
150 ml/5 fl. oz thick béchamel sauce
100 g/4 oz cheddar cheese

## Instructions

1. Preheat the oven to 190°C, 375°F, Gas mark 5 and grease a shallow ovenproof dish.

2. Bring a large pan of salted water to boil, add the cannelloni tubes, and cook for 5–7 minutes or according to the manufacturer's instructions.

3. Meanwhile, heat the butter in a frying pan, add the mushrooms, and sauté for a few minutes until just beginning to soften.

4. Add the mushrooms, peas, and basil to the béchamel sauce and heat gently for 5 minutes, stirring from time to time. Adjust the seasoning.

5. Drain the cannelloni well and stuff with the mushroom mixture. Place in the greased dish, sprinkle with the grated cheese, and bake for 15–20 minutes until brown and bubbling. Serve immediately.

# HAM AND MUSHROOM CANNELLONI

*Notes: Serves 4, main course, hot meal, pork, vegetables, dairy free*

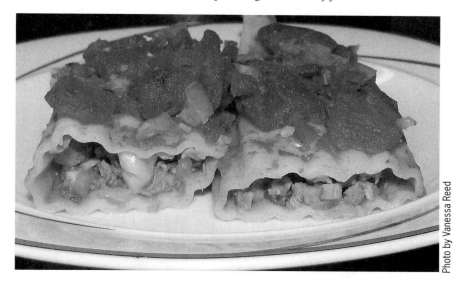

Photo by Vanessa Reed

## Ingredients:

175 g/6 oz mushrooms, *finely chopped*
2 onions, *finely chopped*
1 garlic clove, *crushed*
75 g/3 oz lean ham, *finely chopped*
12 cannelloni tubes
1 x 400 g/14 oz can chopped tomatoes
1 tablespoon tomato purée
1 teaspoon dried mixed herbs

## Instructions

1. Preheat the oven to 200°C, 400°F, Gas mark 6 and grease a shallow ovenproof dish. In a bowl, mix together half the onions, garlic, mushrooms and ham. Divide the stuffing between the cannelloni tubes and place in the ovenproof dish.

2. In a bowl, mix together the chopped tomatoes, tomato purée, and the remaining onions. Spoon over the tubes so that they are all coated. Cover and bake for 25–30 minutes. Serve hot.

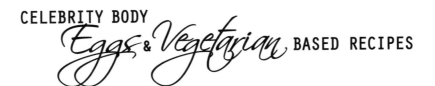

## CHILI OMELET

*Notes: Serves 4, hot meal, vegetarian, main course, gluten, wheat and dairy free*

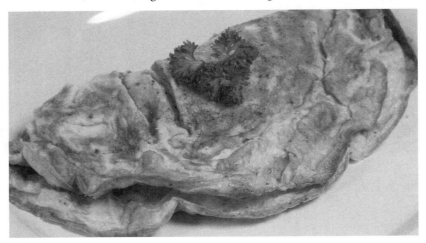

### Ingredients

1 medium onion, *finely sliced*
2 fresh chilies, *deseeded and finely sliced*
1 tablespoon freshly chopped coriander
6 eggs, *beaten*
salt and black pepper
2 tablespoons vegetable oil

### Instructions

1. In a large mixing bowl, mix together the onion, chilies coriander, eggs, salt, and pepper.

2. Heat half the oil in a large frying pan, pour in half the egg mixture, and cook over a medium heat until set. Turn and cook the other side until lightly browned.

3. Remove the cooked omelet from the pan and keep warm while you repeat with the remaining oil and egg mixture.

4. Serve immediately with a fresh tomato sauce.

# CHEESE STUFFED ZUCCHINI

*Notes: Serves 4, hot meal, main course,*
*vegetarian, herbs, gluten and wheat free*

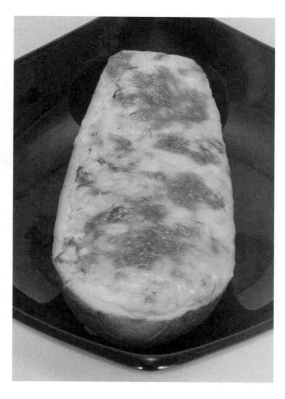

### Ingredients

4 large zucchini
25 g/1oz butter
4 tablespoons onions, *finely chopped*
1 garlic clove, *crushed*
100 g/4 oz double Gloucester cheese
1 egg yolk
1 tablespoon fresh oregano, *chopped*
salt and black pepper

### Instructions

1.  Preheat the oven to 180°C, 350°F,
    Gas mark 4 and grease a shallow
    ovenproof dish. Blanch the zucchini
    in boiling water for 4–5 minutes.
    Remove and cut in half lengthways.
    Scoop out the middle, chop,
    and set aside.

2.  Melt the butter in a saucepan, add the
    onions and garlic, and fry gently for 3–4 minutes, until soft.

3.  Stir in the zucchini, ¾ of the cheese, egg yolk, oregano, and seasoning to
    taste. Divide into 8 and use to fill the zucchini shells.

4.  Arrange in the ovenproof dish, sprinkle with the remaining cheese, and
    bake for 35 minutes, until tender and golden. Serve immediately.

# CHEESE AND ONION QUICHE

*Notes: Serves 4, hot meal, main course, vegetarian, herbs*

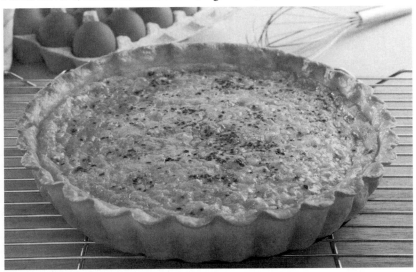

## Ingredients

225 g/8 oz cheese
short crust pastry
4 egg yolks
300 ml/10 fl. oz single cream
2 tablespoons dry vermouth

½ vegetable stock cube
salt and black pepper
grated nutmeg
pinch cayenne pepper
6 tablespoons finely sliced spring onion

## Instructions

1. Heat the oven to 200°C, 400°F, Gas mark 6. Roll out the pastry and line a 22-cm/9-inch flan tin. Prick the pastry bottom with a fork.

2. Line the pastry case with greaseproof and weight it down with dried beans. Bake for 10 minutes. Remove the case from the oven and lift out the paper and beans. Turn the heat down to 150°C, 350°F, Gas mark 4 and return the pastry case for just 5–8 minutes longer, or until the crust is cooked. Brush the case with beaten egg white to seal the crust

3. Meanwhile, beat the egg yolks in a bowl with thin cream until well mixed. Add the stock cube, crumbled, and the dry vermouth. Season with salt, pepper, nutmeg, and cayenne pepper to taste. Stir in the spring onion.

4. Pour the filling into the prepared pastry case and bake for 30–35 minutes. Serve immediately.

There's no magic formula when cooking on a budget. It does take a little planning, creativity, and effort. However, the benefits to your health and your pocket will make the extra effort worthwhile in the long term. If you follow all these tips, beware! You might end up liking this whole economical way of eating so much that when good times return, you won't go back to your old extravagant ways.

# CHAPTER
## *Seven:*
## KEEPING THE FOCUS SHARP 183

# CHAPTER SEVEN:
# KEEPING THE *focus* SHARP

We've all experienced it at some point. You were regularly busting your guts and sweating off your makeup exercising hard. Then, you simply got bored doing the same old thing, listening to the same old thudding tunes on your MP3 player, and found watching the daily news on the TV more exciting. Perhaps you had a terrible bout of flu, which kept you away from your exercise routine. Any progress made is long gone along with all your motivation. Now you'll do anything to avoid exercise.

Even the most dedicated and avid exerciser sometimes flags. Waning motivation, cutting exercise sessions short, and not having your old enthusiasm are all signs of a stale exercise regimen. What's to be done? The more you procrastinate, the worse you feel, but the thought of being flabby and sagging is potentially too intimidating.

It's well documented that even small amounts of exercise can make a difference, as people are anxious to begin some type of workout or exercise routine. Often people will jump in and, after a few weeks or months, get frustrated and find themselves back in their old routines. Exercise can often prove to be hard work, especially when other life considerations get in the way. Whether you're a seasoned exercise veteran or someone who is just beginning to exercise, finding the right motivation at the right time can be critical to your success.

The hard part will be to continue exercising. When you're tired, stressed, or busy, that is when you need to exercise the most. Besides being a great stress reliever, exercise can make you sleep better and clear your head for more productivity during the day.

What you do to keep motivated is often just as important to you as why you began to exercise. The key is to remember that you need to find what works for you. You must find your own motivation, deep inside of yourself. There is no other source of motivation because if you aren't willing to do the work, then nothing else will make you. Exercise motivation is unique to each person. Your motivation to do something is the reason why you want to do it. If you have motivation, you do something because you want to do it, and not because you have to do it.

## CONSIDER THIS:

One way to stay motivated is to constantly remind yourself that a worthwhile payoff lies ahead—a new, healthy, strong you is emerging. Effective, consistent exercise will not only improve your overall health and fitness, but it will also improve your appearance, energy level, and social interactions. Also, look forward to the many psychological benefits of exercise as well: confidence, self-esteem, and relief from depression, anxiety, and stress.

If you are serious about your health and well-being, you will take action and stick with an exercise program, and you will benefit in all these ways. Once you see the results, you will become even more motivated. Action creates motivation!

Your first plan of action is to make exercise a habit again. It takes on average three weeks to develop a routine. While a three times a week workout of twenty minutes each is the prescribed minimum, you might find a light daily workout better for getting back into the habit. Start off exercising three or more times a week for twenty minutes or more, and work up to at least thirty minutes, four to six times a week. This can include several short bouts of activity in a day. Take a close look at your program and determine what's causing your exercise stagnation. Then use my ideas on how to inject life back into your routine.

## SET GOALS FOR MOTIVATION

Goal setting is another great way of staying motivated. Goals focus your workout program and clarify what you are trying to achieve. As you attain each goal, you gain encouragement and further motivation. Here is how to achieve the goals you set and obtain the results you deserve:

1. **MAKE SURE YOUR GOALS ARE MEASURABLE.** A vague goal, such as "I want to be fit," gives you little to aim for. Decide when and what you are going to achieve, such as "I want to lose 2 percent of my body fat by the time I get married."

2. **BE REALISTIC.** Make sure your goals are attainable. If you set your expectations too high, you will get frustrated and will be more likely to quit. Make sure, however, that your goals are not too easy. They should be challenging. When you achieve a challenging goal, your pride and satisfaction will generate more motivation.

3. **SET SHORT-TERM GOALS AS STEPPINGSTONES TO YOUR "ULTIMATE" (LONG-TERM) GOALS.** If your long-term goal is to lose 10 pounds in one year, then set short-term weekly or monthly goals to achieve your long-term goal. Develop a plan. It is a lot easier to accomplish a goal one day, one week, or one month at a time, such as losing a half pound a week, than it is to think that you need to decrease your weight by 10 pounds.

## MAKE IT FUN

Another way of assuring that you stay motivated is to make exercise fun. If you perceive your workout as a chore, you're more than likely to not stick with it. Here are some techniques for making your workout something to look forward to:

1. **ADD VARIETY.** If your exercises are getting tedious and boring, change one of these factors:

   ~ Vary how often you do an exercise and the number of sets and reps you do.

   ~ Find an alternate exercise. For example, if you always do leg squats using dumbbells, try doing it with a resistance band. Change the order of the exercises you do for each muscle group and the muscle groups themselves.

2. **INCLUDE FRIENDS AND FAMILY.** Training with a workout partner not only makes your training session more fun, safe, and intense, but it also increases the likelihood of your showing up for your workouts. Make sure you pick a partner whose goals and interests are similar to yours and who is willing to spot you correctly and motivate you to do your best.

3. **FIGHT DISCOURAGEMENT.** If once in a long while you skip a workout because you choose to go out with friends, just accept and enjoy your choice. Try not to feel guilty. Otherwise, the sense of failure can make it harder to get yourself back on track. Focus on how much progress you have made so far, not on how far you have to go.

4. **EXPECT AND PREPARE FOR PLATEAUS.** If you feel you have reached a plateau and/or are bored, don't give up. This is a natural process of your exercise plan. Make sure to vary the exercises, sets, repetitions, and order of your workout. Continually search for new ways of making your routine fun and exciting.

## KEEP TRACK OF YOUR PROGRESS

1. **SCHEDULE YOUR WORKOUT.** If you always exercise on the same days at the same time, your routine will become a fixture in your life, not a whim. Missing a training session will begin to feel unnatural. Including exercise into your busy schedule will be an adjustment, and staying motivated will be equally challenging. Change is difficult for many people. However, if you have the willingness to work through the initial emotional discomfort as you move step by step through a safe and effective program, you will find the confidence, commitment, and determination that will ease the way.

2. **AFTER YOU SET YOUR GOALS AND WRITE THEM DOWN, YOU WANT TO ALSO CHART YOUR PROGRESS.** Be sure to write down your daily achievements to compare to your goals. This will become extremely motivating as you see yourself meeting your goals. With consistent exercise, you will also see your workouts becoming easier and your ability to work harder and longer growing. This often happens faster than visible results on your body, such as weight loss or definition. Many people become frustrated and quit exercise right before big changes are about to happen because they don't see the results on their bodies. Seeing measurable progress on paper will keep you motivated while you work toward the bigger goals you have set for yourself. Photocopy and make use of the Personal Progress Chart in this book and start logging your progress as suggested.

## BE ACCOUNTABLE!

About 95 percent of all participants in an exercise program will stop exercising. Why? No support. It's a fact that exercisers with some kind of support system have a better chance of continuing exercise.

You need someone who will also hold you accountable for your exercise. Working with someone like a personal trainer, a willing partner, or a mentor will give you the support you need, and you can work together to identify barriers to keeping your commitment and develop strategies to overcome these obstacles. Most people need far more support, follow up, and accountability than they think to start and maintain an exercise program.

## GET OBJECTIVE FEEDBACK

You may know what a good workout feels like—you have that endorphin "high" after exercise, or you have energy to spare all day long. But do you know what an effective workout feels like? It is hard to know how effective your workout is every day without waiting for weeks or months to see the results. What if you could see day after day how many calories you burned, or what your heart rate was each workout? Using a heart rate monitor can tell you if you are working too hard or not hard enough. What about calories? A heart rate monitor can tell you all day long how many calories you are burning and keep you motivated to move! When you look for ways to add activity to your day, it becomes a fun game and you can instantly see the results.

## AVOID THE 'ALL-OR-NOTHING' APPROACH

Have you had plans to exercise five times one week and the first day something happened and you didn't exercise? When this happens, many people give up on the rest of the week. This is known as the all-or-nothing mentality. Avoid this at all cost—it doesn't work. If you approach your exercise and nutrition program in that manner, you set yourself up for failure. Allow for flexibility in your exercise plans and know one missed day is not a setback.

In the interest of avoiding the all-or-nothing mentality, don't try to implement all these secrets at once. Pick one or two, and when you have those working, add another secret. Just like results from exercise, building motivation and consistency will take time. Fitness is not just about reaching a destination, it is a journey where you will learn much about yourself and grow from your experiences. Keep your short-term goals in mind, and enjoy the journey to reaching your ultimate goals.

# PERSONAL PROGRESS CHART

The key to reaching your goals with the *Celebrity Body on a Budget* workout plans is consistency. Charting your progress is an effective and invaluable way of helping you to adhere to a program correctly and remain motivated. It would be a good idea to make several photocopies of this personal progress chart and use it to record your exercise and eating habits. I've designed this user-friendly chart to make record keeping as easy as possible—after all I'm sure you'd rather spend your valuable time doing your workout plan than sitting and writing about it!

So that you can log your progress using this chart, there are three main headings. An example is given in the first column of the chart. From there, it's up to you to start being honest with yourself and fill in this chart on a daily or weekly basis. Good luck.

## PERSONAL PROGRESS CHART

|  | Example | Week 1 | Week 2 | Week 3 | Week 4 | Week 5 | Week 6 |
|---|---|---|---|---|---|---|---|
| **Number of Workouts for the Week** | | | | | | | |
| Exercise Neophyte | 2 | | | | | | |
| Progressive Exerciser | 3 | | | | | | |
| Adventurous Exerciser | 4 | | | | | | |
| Specialist Exerciser | 5 | | | | | | |

| | Example | Week 1 | Week 2 | Week 3 | Week 4 | Week 5 | Week 6 |
|---|---|---|---|---|---|---|---|
| **How You Felt During the Week** | | | | | | | |
| Exhausted | | | | | | | |
| Fairly Tired | | | | | | | |
| Irritable/ Moody | | | | | | | |
| Bored | | | | | | | |
| Relaxed | | | | | | | |
| Fine | | | | | | | |
| Energized | Yes | | | | | | |
| In Control | | | | | | | |
| **How You Felt Before Your Exercise Session** | | | | | | | |
| Tired | Yes | | | | | | |
| Reluctant | Yes | | | | | | |
| Lacking Motivation | Yes | | | | | | |
| Rearing to Go | | | | | | | |
| **How You Felt During Your Exercise Session** | | | | | | | |
| All Exercises Were Tough | | | | | | | |
| Some Exercises Were Hard | Yes | | | | | | |
| Comfortable | | | | | | | |
| Exercises Were Easy | | | | | | | |
| I Could Do More | | | | | | | |
| **How You Felt After the Exercise Session** | | | | | | | |
| Invigorated | Yes | | | | | | |
| Fine | | | | | | | |
| Tired | | | | | | | |
| Exhausted | | | | | | | |

| | Example | Week 1 | Week 2 | Week 3 | Week 4 | Week 5 | Week 6 |
|---|---|---|---|---|---|---|---|
| **Indicate Your Eating Habits** | | | | | | | |
| Controlled | Yes | | | | | | |
| Well Planned | Yes | | | | | | |
| Hopeless | | | | | | | |
| Binged | | | | | | | |
| Increased Fruit Intake | Yes | | | | | | |
| Decreased Fruit Intake | | | | | | | |
| Increased Vegetable Intake | Yes | | | | | | |
| Decreased Vegetable Intake | | | | | | | |
| Increased Water Intake | Yes | | | | | | |
| Decreased Water Intake | | | | | | | |
| Increased Fat Intake | | | | | | | |
| Reduced Fat Intake | Yes | | | | | | |
| Ate Take-out | 2 | | | | | | |
| Excess Sugar Intake | | | | | | | |
| Lowered Sugar Intake | Yes | | | | | | |
| Excess Dairy Products | | | | | | | |
| Lowered Dairy Products | Yes | | | | | | |
| **How You Feel About What You've Managed to Achieve During the Week** | | | | | | | |
| Failed Miserably | | | | | | | |
| Achieved Little | | | | | | | |
| Achieved Most of My Goals | Yes | | | | | | |
| Achieved All of My Goals and More | | | | | | | |

# CHAPTER *Eight:*

CHAPTER EIGHT:

# EVERYTHING YOU *always* WANTED TO KNOW ABOUT EXERCISE, FITNESS AND DIET (WELL ALMOST!)

Making healthy choices that fit your lifestyle, so you can do the things you want to do, is the first step in achieving and maintaining a fit, lean, and healthy body. Since many people have the same concerns about exercise and weight management, you'll probably have many questions as you progress through this book. Take a look at answers from this book to the most frequently asked questions and myths about fitness and diet.

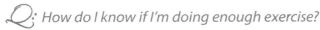 *How do I know if I'm doing enough exercise?*

**ANSWER:** If you are exercising for health reasons (to reduce heart disease, reduce stress or diabetes, for example), complete five to six days a week of moderate-paced walking, getting slightly out of breath. Going shopping or gardening is not sufficient enough. If exercising for fitness, complete a minimum of thirty minutes of exercise at 60 percent to 90 percent of your maximum heart rate five times a week, introducing one set of eight to ten reps of strength exercises for major muscle groups. If you are overweight and need to reduce excess weight, aim for sixty to ninety minutes per day of moderate-intensity walking. If you're past fifty years of age, more emphasis needs to be placed on strength, mobility, and balance, as loss of these directly affect your physical independence.

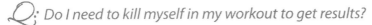 *Do I need to kill myself in my workout to get results?*

**ANSWER:** Intensity is one key to successful exercise. For your body to adapt and improve, you have to challenge it. Some avid exercisers take this too far. Interval training, which is high intensity cardio training, is one of the most effective ways to raise your metabolism and burn more fat. The problem happens when people do high intensity all the time. Your body needs rest to improve and overdoing high intensity exercise overtrains the body and your performance declines. The key is to constantly progress your exercise program with balance, proper nutrition, and adequate rest.

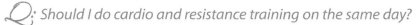

**Q:** *Should I do cardio and resistance training on the same day?*

**ANSWER:** Your cardio and strength workouts utilize energy from two different energy systems. The two most common energy systems that your body uses are your aerobic and anaerobic metabolisms. Because you burn energy differently, you can do cardio and strength training on the same day; however, I recommend that you do high-intensity cardio on its own day. You do use some anaerobic energy in the first couple minutes of a cardio session so it is ideal to do weights before cardio, as anaerobic energy is the main energy source during resistance training.

**Q:** *When is the best time to work out? Is it good for your body to exercise at night before you go to sleep?*

**ANSWER:** Any time during the day is appropriate for exercise, but you should schedule your workout around your eating patterns. Don't exercise right after eating; give yourself an hour for digestion before exercising. At the same time, avoid eating for forty-five minutes after exercise to burn your body fat. The most important thing is that you need to exercise for a healthy body, and if you find it hard to take out time to exercise in the morning, then evening is a good option.

It must have been past one hour before you have eating something and at the same time you need to keep yourself off food for another 45 min after exercise to burn your body fat.

**Q:** *Does muscle burn more calories than fat?*

**ANSWER:** Muscle is metabolically active, living tissue while about 90 percent of fat tissue is triglyceride, or oil, and is inert tissue. Once you begin exercising, you have started the process of developing lean muscle. By increasing lean muscle, you'll burn more calories than fat, even when you're sleeping. After training, muscles require a large amount of calories to rebuild and recover. That means that an active person with more muscle mass burns more calories just sitting than does an inactive person with less muscle. Also bear in mind that muscle weighs more than fat so don't get discouraged if you're exercising regularly and not losing weight. Dump your scales in favor of how your clothes fit and feel.

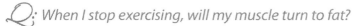

*Q: When I stop exercising, will my muscle turn to fat?*

**ANSWER:** Muscles can't and won't turn to fat. When you exercise, your muscles become more dense and stronger because exercise causes extra protein building blocks, called amino acids, to deposit in the muscles. If you cease exercising, fewer amino acids go into your muscles so the muscles decrease in size. Your body has no way to store extra protein, so amino acids that are not used in your muscles are picked up by your liver, which uses them for energy or converts them into fat for storage. So if you stop exercising, you simply eat less or you'll gain weight. But muscles never turn into fat.

*Q: What are some things that I can measure to see if I'm making any improvements?*

**ANSWER:** You could keep track of your:

A. **Resting heart rate (RHR):** A stronger, more efficient heart will have a lower RHR.

B. **Body measurements:** Measure your hips, waist, thighs, and calves (and anything else you may want to keep track of). If you need to lose body fat, these measurements will decrease gradually as you lose fat. Bear in mind that at the same time, hopefully, you are gaining muscle.

C. **Rate of perceived exertion (RPE):** As you become more fit, your RPE for a specific exercise may change. For example, if you've been sedentary and start a program of walking for a month, your RPE will most likely be higher for the walk on your first day of the program compared to the walk on your last day for the same distance and pace.

D. **Clothes, jewelry:** If you are trying to lose body fat, you may notice looseness in your clothing or in jewelry such as rings or watches.

E. **Weight:** Anecdotally, this seems to be the last thing to rely on. You may only notice a decrease in weight after seeing other improvements in your body.

*Q: Can I exercise too much?*

**ANSWER**: Definitely. More is not necessarily better. Beginners should take a rest day at least every other day, while those who are more active should consider taking a rest day after a vigorous workout or alternate exercise programs so that you're working different muscle groups. You must give your body a chance to recover from the stress of exercising. Some signs of too much exercise could include: chronic fatigue, decrease in performance, increase in recovery requirements, altered resting heart rate, and muscle soreness and damage. Not everyone will have these symptoms. Listen to your body. If you're not feeling well, consult a doctor and mention the intensity and frequency of your workouts.

*Q: I've no time for exercise and don't really like it, what can I do?*

**ANSWER:** Alter your perception of exercise being purely about gyms and getting hot and sweaty. Instead, use the ideas in this book to your advantage and think accumulated physical activity. Invest in a heart rate monitor with a built-in pedometer (or acquire them separately) and go walking. Establish your baseline daily steps, increasing this by 2,500 steps a week at a time. Aim to consolidate this daily until you're achieving over 7,500 steps a day. If you partake in fewer than 4,500 steps a day, this defines you as being sedentary. A highly active individual consistently accumulates more than 12,500 steps daily. Use this as a springboard for motivation and to feel positive about your efforts in your available time.

*Q: I'm a woman, and I want to start weight training.*
*Will I get big, bulging muscles from doing this?*

**ANSWER:** If it is your desire to build large lean muscle tissue through specific weight training, then it's highly probable. To create muscle mass, you must perform large amounts of sets on each muscle group every week. The average of two to four sets per body part every other day is not enough total volume to ever get anyone bulky or big. Also, to build mass you need to consume vast amounts of calories. A bodybuilder may eat up to 8,000 calories in a day to create his or her large physique. A well-balanced exercise plan will enable you to create a fitter and leaner body that's firm and toned. Remember, too, the many benefits of weight training: It will increase your muscle, and muscle burns more calories than fat. Resistance exercise, such as free weights; weight training machines; or exercise bands can affect bone mass, which can help prevent osteoporosis.

*Q: I do tons of sit-ups and still have a stubborn pot belly. How do I get a flatter stomach or a six-pack?*

**ANSWER:** Many people think sit-ups and crunches are the only exercises you can do for the stomach. Sit-ups are effective for training your outer stomach muscles, which will mainly work the upper abs but will not actually draw the stomach in if worked on their own. The secret to six-pack abs is total body fitness. Performing an abundance of crunches will not raise your metabolism high enough to burn enough fat away from your abs. A good aerobic training program and a core total body fitness strength program will burn the most total amounts of fat and give you the best abs. A well-rounded fitness plan involving utilizing your core muscles, which keep your abs engaged throughout the movements, will encourage better looking abs. You'll see a flatter stomach in no time.

*Q: What can I do to tone up my flabby "bat wing" arms?*

**ANSWER:** As we age, our skin loses elasticity and becomes less able to support the natural layer of fat underneath it. This causes the fat to drop, giving the appearance of jowls in the face and flabby underarms. While you can't do anything to dramatically alter the elasticity of the skin, you can train to get your arms as lean as possible, which would decrease the amount of hanging fat and tone the muscle underneath the fat layers. Doing lots of low-medium intensity cardiovascular exercise of thirty to sixty minutes, three times a week, might help to burn away the fat from under the arms. Also, cutting out high sugar foods and saturated fats will go a long way to helping you achieve your results. Train the triceps muscles by doing exercises such as tricep extensions and dips for two sets of twelve to fifteen repetitions.

*Q: Can I spot reduce a specific area?*

**ANSWER:** In general, the answer is no. You lose fat throughout the body. Normally, the face is one of the first places people lose fat. Most people have a trouble area, which is an area where their body stores more fat. If you are having a problem losing your gut or love handles, it is probably because you are doing something every day to store more fat. Often, people who exercise and eat well still have a bad habit that slows their metabolism and stores fat each day. This is seen where you are losing weight though it never seems to leave your belly.

***Q:*** *I work out and eat healthily, but my weight just plateaus. Why?*

**ANSWER:** It's highly probable that you're gaining muscle, especially if you have increased your resistance training. Keep things in perspective, and assess your body shape with a tape measure as well as with the weighing scales. Avoid your body getting complacent by varying your workouts in terms of both activity and intensity. Boost calorie expenditure with interval training of varied-pace bouts. Also consider how physically active you are outside your exercise sessions, particularly when at work (see the section on Office Workouts). If you are sedentary most of the time, then you are expecting a lot of weight change from what could effectively be just three hourly workouts a week.

***Q:*** *How do I stop my middle spreading?*

**ANSWER:** Changes in hormones and long-term chronic stress contribute to body fat around the middle. These changes put individuals over forty-five years of age at a higher risk of cardiovascular disease, so establish good health habits now. Effective abdominal exercises will help, but boosting your regular cardiovascular activity for thirty to forty-five minutes, five to six days a week, needs to be a priority. This helps reduce the stress hormone cortisol and significantly decreases cardiovascular risks associated with a spreading mid region. With abdominal exercises, make sure you have a good technique because straining can exacerbate a protruding belly.

***Q:*** *My legs aren't fat, but they lack definition.*
*How do I make them shapelier?*

**ANSWER:** The best exercises to do for all-over leg definition are exercises that use all the major leg muscles in one go. Squats and lunges are all excellent leg exercises that will improve your leg definition if done slowly two to four times per week. By doing these major muscle group exercises not only will you improve leg definition, but due to the size of the muscles, you will burn plenty of calories, too. You will also be impressed by how quickly you can increase the number of squats and lunges you can do in one session.

**Q:** *If I burn 3,500 calories, will I burn off one pound of fat?*

**ANSWER:** One pound of fat is worth 3,500 calories to the body. However, if you just burn 3,500 calories, you won't necessarily lose a pound of fat. When you burn calories, you never just burn fat. You constantly burn carbohydrates and fat combined every day. The key is to raise your metabolism so you burn more calories all day long.

**Q:** *What is cross training?*

**ANSWER:** Cross training is simply an exercise program that involves more than one mode of training. Combining strength, cardio, and flexibility training can allow different parts of the body to develop. It also lets you rest muscles and bones without needing to stop training. This allows better all round fitness to develop and also provides a little variety to maintain your motivation.

**Q:** *I've been overweight most of my life.*
*Are my genes responsible for me being overweight?*

**ANSWER:** It's highly probable that your genetic predisposition will have some influence on your body weight and its shape. There are some genetic complications that may help contribute to difficulty in losing weight such as hormone imbalance, certain enzyme deficiencies, or problems with the cell energy pathways. However, it has been estimated that genetic disorders account for less than 5 percent in obese people. Many people just exercise too little and eat too much.

**Q:** *Are women naturally fatter than men?*

**ANSWER:** Women do tend to have more weight problems than men, but that may be because women tend to have a naturally higher body fat percentage. Men usually have more lean body weight, which results in a higher metabolic rate.

*Q: What are some warning signs I should look for while exercising?*

**ANSWER:** You should immediately stop exercising if you feel unusual pain, such as pain in your left or mid-chest area or left neck, shoulder, or arm during or just after exercising. Also take note if you experience a sudden lightness in your head, cold sweats, or fainting. These might not be the only signs your body will give you. Other signs can include headache, dizziness, nausea, and muscular or joint pain. Always remember to listen to your body—no one knows your body better than you!

*Q: What is the pain in my side that occurs without warning while I am exercising?*

**ANSWER:** This pain is commonly called a side stitch or just a "stitch" for short. The cause of a stitch is debated, but it is likely to be related to stressing the ligaments between the diaphragm and the stomach. Generally, a stitch is nothing to do with what you have eaten. To avoid a stitch, which is often a severe pain, know your limitations and do not push yourself too hard. If you experience a stitch, then try to alleviate the pain by breathing deeply, bending forward, or simply lowering the pace of your workout.

*Q: Is exercising when I am experiencing pain okay?*

**ANSWER:** That all depends on where the pain is, how long you have had it, and whether you know how it was caused. Pain is the body warning you about something, but a light degree of soreness for a day or two after rigorous exercise is to be expected. If you know exactly how you caused the pain, then it makes it easier to determine whether you should worry about it or not. For example, if you know a specific exercise caused a worrying pain, then you should refrain from that exercise and then later on analyze the technique you used and alter it accordingly. What is concerning is a pain that is so bad it disrupts your life, such as keeps you from walking or hinders your sleep. This could be an injury that will be aggravated by further exercise, so consult a physiotherapist or your doctor. Other signs that your pain signifies an injury include if the pain is localized, if there is swelling in the affected area, if the pain persists for longer than a week, or if the pain gets progressively worse instead of better. Pain in your joints is also cause for concern. In any of these cases, rest your body and consult your doctor.

*Q: Is profuse sweating during exercise a sign that I am not fit enough?*

**ANSWER:** Not at all, it is the body's natural way of cooling itself down. It will be more evident when you're exercising in a hot and humid environment. Different individuals sweat varying amounts. Some would argue that if you don't sweat, then you're not exercising hard enough! It is nothing to be concerned about.

*Q: Is it true that people who exercise regularly live longer and visit the doctor less frequently than those who don't?*

**ANSWER:** Many studies show that people who exercise regularly live longer than those who lead an inactive life. Exercise seems to reduce the risk and severity of some potentially life-threatening conditions, while helping people to stay active well into their later years. Of course, a long and healthy life is also determined by genetics, nutrition, environment, and stress—but your own efforts can make a difference. Even a little exercise is better than none, and you do not have to spend all your leisure hours exercising.

Studies show that gentle walking, climbing stairs, cycling at a moderate pace, and other active recreational pursuits help people to stay healthier and more alert, and to outlive their sedentary counterparts.

*Q: How many calories should I eat every day in order to lose weight fast?*

**ANSWER:** This is the most frequently asked weight loss question ever, and the truth is that total calories consumed each day is not the most important factor. Rather, the amount of food eaten at any one sitting is what determines whether you will gain weight or lose weight. Too much emphasis has been placed on "calories per day" according to a person's height and weight. This is now known to be false because it is "calories per meal" that determines whether your body will burn those calories or store them as fat tissue. For example, you could eat 2,500 calories spread out evenly all day and lose more weight than if you starved yourself all day and then ate a 2,000-calorie dinner. Instead of concentrating on calories per day, focus on what you eat at each individual sitting.

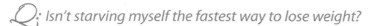

*Q: Isn't starving myself the fastest way to lose weight?*

**ANSWER:** Many people believe that since overeating is responsible for weight gain, then "starving" must be the quickest way to lose weight. Sounds logical at first, after all, since 3,500 calories equals one pound and the quickest way to get rid of 3,500 calories is to starve. The fact is, however, that the more you starve yourself, the fewer calories your body begins burning each day. So if your body was formerly burning 3,000 calories per day and you begin starving yourself, then your body will adjust and soon begin burning only 2,000 calories per day, then perhaps 1,500 calories per day, and if you starve yourself enough, it will burn even fewer calories than that until you will be starving yourself and burning few calories at all.

*Q: How much water should I drink each day in order to lose weight?*

**ANSWER:** Many people have been told to drink as much water as they can consume each day and that somehow this will miraculously speed up the weight loss process. The plain fact is that it's important to drink water each day because water helps your body in many ways. But you will not gain some magical advantage to losing weight by drinking gallons of water per day. Water is important in any diet, but if you're drinking so much water that the thought of another glass makes you feel "sick," then you have already consumed enough and you won't be getting any advantage by forcing another glass of water on yourself.

*Q: If I eat all low-fat and fat-free foods will I lose weight?*

**ANSWER:** It is now a widely known fact that the consumption of excess carbohydrates is one of the quickest ways to gain weight, and the likes of the Atkins diet and Zone diet are proof of that fact.

In fact, many low-fat and fat-free foods have so many excess carbohydrates (to replace the missing fat) that they can make you gain extraordinary amounts of weight by eating them too often or in excessive quantities. Eating low fat is always a good idea compared to gorging yourself on fatty foods, but relying solely on low-fat foods will not solve your weight problems. It takes a careful balance between fat and carbohydrates (and exercise) to begin losing weight at the fastest and safest rate.

*Q: What types of food should I eat before exercising?*
*How long before exercising should I eat?*

**ANSWER:** Carbohydrates are important to maintain blood-glucose levels during exercise, and protein levels are slightly increased in highly active people. It is recommended that you eat a meal or snack, preferably low in fat and fiber, before exercising to provide sufficient fluid to maintain hydration during exercising.

*Q: How do I lose five to ten pounds a week?*

**ANSWER:** It is unrealistic to hope to lose that amount of weight so quickly. If you set a goal like this, you will set yourself up for failure. A far more realistic goal is losing one to two pounds per week. You need to simply burn more calories than you eat. To lose one pound a week, you need to burn 500 calories more than you eat each day. Don't be fooled by the misinformation freely available everywhere. There isn't a miracle pill. Exercise machines aren't the complete solution. Eliminating carbohydrates isn't the answer.

*Q: What should I do if I hit a plateau*
*during the course of losing weight?*

**ANSWER:** Hitting a plateau during any weight loss program is normal. Your body requires fewer calories to function as your weight decreases. Everyone's body levels off at a different weight. Some people will level off at a higher weight than others.

Gradually increasing the amount or intensity of your physical activity may help you continue to lose, while for others it will help to maintain their new weight. Even a modest weight loss of 5 percent to 10 percent with maintenance can provide important health benefits. Any activity that gets you moving helps you on the way to a healthy lifestyle.

*Are there any foods or supplements that will
help me burn more calories?*

**ANSWER:** Generally, the answer is no. Contrary to the claims of some diets, there are no foods that increase your body's ability to burn calories. There are foods, spices, and supplements that cause a little more increase in heat than other foods, but exercise and diet are the key ingredients. There is no magic pill that will enable you to shed the fat that has taken you years to put on.

*Do you recommend eating five or six small meals a day
rather than three large ones?*

**ANSWER:** Our bodies do very well with grazing. Your body adapts to the smaller meals, so you tend to want less food. Also you can burn those calories more efficiently. If you have a large meal, the amount of insulin rises to a higher level. When insulin is high, it turns off the fat-release enzyme called hormone-sensitive lipase, so it takes a much longer time to burn off and utilize fat. If you have a smaller meal, you can utilize the fat a lot more efficiently. Stick with the smaller, more regular meals for better weight control.

*Once I have completed the challenges in this book,
how do I maintain my level of fitness?*

**ANSWER:** With *Celebrity Body on a Budget* there is not an "end" to the program because it evolves with you. If you feel you have achieved all your original goals, then feel free to reprofile yourself, but for most people there is no need to do that. The best way to maintain your results is to maintain your program. It's as simple as that. However, the biggest thing to remember is that it takes time to see significant changes.
So don't expect major physical changes over night. Set a goal and work toward that.

# CHAPTER
## *Nine:*
## LEARN MORE TO EARN MORE

# LEARN MORE TO *earn* MORE

## FITNESS AND HEALTHY EATING RESOURCES

**www.cmcfit.co.uk**—Read about the author with pictures of celebrity clients

**www.doitforcharity.com/home**—The largest Web site in the United Kingdom for charity events. Why not blend a fitness challenge with a great cause and make a difference for yourself and others?

**www.nhs.uk/Change4Life**—Government-funded campaign to create public awareness of the benefits of healthy lifestyle changes.

**www.nutrition.org.uk**—Provides healthy eating information, resources for schools, news items, recipes, and details of this organization's work around the world.

## EXERCISE EQUIPMENT AND CLOTHING RESOURCES

**www.sportsworkout.com**—World-renowned sport-specific fitness, strength, and conditioning online personal training site. This company offers fitness and nutrition books and DVDs, exercise equipment, and over 1,700 discount nutritional supplements.

**www.fitness-superstore.co.uk**—The largest supplier of fitness equipment in the United Kingdom, offering the best possible prices on all fitness equipment with delivery across the UK in the fastest possible time.

**www.hirefitness.co.uk**—The ideal solution if your business or family commitments make it difficult for you to visit the gym or you simply would prefer to work out at home. This company offers try before you buy options on exercise equipment.

**www.heartratemonitor.co.uk**—The team behind BHIP Ltd. has been selling heart rate monitors online from since 1999. BHIP is recognized as the undisputed online leader in heart rate monitors.

**www.sweatybetty.com**—Top fitness clothing retailers who push the boundaries on product and styling.

# FITNESS AND DIET MAGAZINES AND BOOKS RESOURCES

Physical and online bookstores—Look for other fitness titles written by the author including Triple A Fitness Program for Anyone, Anywhere, Anytime (published by Quadrille) and Bone Idle to Body Idol (Get a Life!) (published by Hodder).

**www.womensfitness.co.uk**—Women's complete guide to healthy living.

**www.mensfitness.com**—World-renowned men's fitness magazine.

# ENERGY EXPENDITURE CHART

Use the calorie expenditure chart on the next page to calculate the approximate number of calories burned when performing various activities. The calorie expenditure chart lists activities in order of effort starting with the easier movements progressing down toward the higher energy activities. If the calorie expenditure chart does not list your activity, then try comparing it to an activity listed which closely resembles the same level of effort. For example, skating is fairly close to brisk walking in the amount of effort required so the calories burned will be about the same. This is the easiest way to find the best calorie burning exercise to help you lose weight.

## A. SEDENTARY ACTIVITIES ENERGY COSTS — CALORIES/HOUR*

| | |
|---|---|
| Lying down or sleeping | 90 |
| Sitting quietly | 84 |
| Sitting and writing, card playing, etc. | 114 |

## B. MODERATE ACTIVITIES (150-350)

| | |
|---|---|
| Bicycling (5 mph) | 174 |
| Canoeing (2.5 mph) | 174 |
| Dancing (ballroom) | 210 |
| Golf (twosome, carrying clubs) | 324 |
| Horseback riding (sitting to trot) | 246 |
| Light housework, cleaning, etc. | 246 |
| Swimming (crawl, 20 yards/minute) | 288 |
| Tennis (recreational doubles) | 312 |
| Volleyball (recreational) | 264 |
| Walking (2 mph) | 198 |

## C. VIGOROUS ACTIVITIES (MORE THAN 350)

| | |
|---|---|
| Aerobic dancing | 546 |
| Basketball (recreational) | 450 |
| Bicycling (13 mph) | 612 |
| Circuit training | 756 |
| (Celebrity Body on a Budget Workout) | |
| Football (touch, vigorous) | 498 |
| Ice Skating (9 mph) | 384 |
| Racquetball | 588 |
| Roller skating (9 mph) | 384 |
| Jogging (10-minute mile, 6 mph) | 654 |
| Scrubbing floors | 440 |
| Swimming (crawl, 45 yards/minute) | 522 |
| Tennis (recreational singles) | 450 |
| Cross-country skiing ( 5 mph) | 690 |

*Hourly estimates based on values calculated for calories burned per minute for a 150 pound person.*

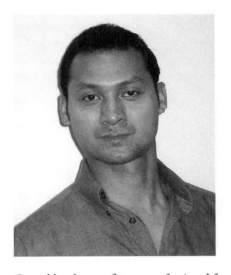

Cornel Chin is a high-profile fitness expert to the stars. Cornel integrates his diverse background to create an all-encompassing approach to fitness. As a leading fitness expert, he is a frequent guest on numerous television and radio shows. Cornel has also featured in, and regularly contributes to, a host of leading international publications. He is also the author of *Exercise for Everyone* (published by Quadrille Publishing Ltd., 2004), and *Bone Idle to Body Idol* (published by Hodder, 2006), which are both endorsed by his celebrity clients.

Cornel has been a fitness professional for more than seventeen years and is credited for getting Leonardo DiCaprio into shape in double quick time for the film *The Beach;* Colin Firth for the film *Bridget Jones's Diary;* Audrey Tautou, star of the film *Da Vinci Code* and *Amélie;* Tilda Swinton, star of *The Chronicles of Narnia;* and Naomie Harris, of *Miami Vice* and *Pirates of the Caribbean* fame. Other celebrity clients include actor Joseph Fiennes *(Shakespeare In Love)*, pop star Rick Astley, actress Virginie LeDoyen, actor Paterson Joseph, actress Victoria Smurfit, Sir Terry Farrell OBE CBE (world-renowned architect), actress Raquel Cassidy, and Deborah Moore (daughter of actor Roger Moore).

As the owner of his own fitness consultancy, Cornel offers personal training services, instructor workshops, seminars, product endorsement, and is expanding his horizons to include more health and fitness television productions. He is currently developing a number of portable exercise devices.

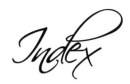
# Index

## K

**Knee-ups,** *marching, 100*

## L

**Lifestyle,** *changes, 48, 207*

**Location of home gym,** *54*

**Low impact:**
*exercise, 60*
*workout, 58-59*

**Lunges:**
*360-degree, 129*
*alternate forward, 119*
*alternate side leg, 106*
*jump, 146*
*weighted, 93*

## M

**Measure:**
*cardiovascular endurance, 77*
*endurance, 82*
*flexibility, 17*
*heart rate, 18, 75*
*strength, 82*

**Measurements:**
*body, 195*
*weight, 71*

**Medical condition,** *54, 93*

**Mesomorph,** *11-12, 15*

**Motivation,** *28, 33, 183-184,*
*187, 189, 196, 199*

**Multigyms,** *53*

**Muscle:**
*building, 14, 57, 89*
*conditioning, 92-93, 207*
*contractions, 9, 17, 64*
*tissue, 9*
*tone, 1, 14, 31, 61, 89*

**Muscles:**
*abdominal, 132, 149, 151, 153*
*back, 26-27*
*balancing, 30*
*buttock, 27, 43*
*flexor, 82*
*gluteus, 24*

*leg, 84, 198*
*shoulder, 17, 26*
*skeletal, 9*
*stomach, 77, 126, 139, 144, 152, 197*
*thigh, 98*
*tummy, 108, 114*
*voluntary, 9*

**Muscular system,** *function*
*of, 9*

## N

**Nutrition:**
*basic, 162*
*books and DVDs, 207*
*fact label, 162*
*proper, 193*

## O

**Oblique crunches,** *24*

**Office:**
*desk, 35*
*exercises, 33-34, 48*

**Osteoperosis,** *62, 196*

**Overhead press,** *110*

**Overweight,** *166-167, 193, 199*

## P

**Pain:**
*back, 58*
*free stretch, 9*
*reduce, 62*
*localized, 200*
*when is it okay?, 200*

**PCr,** *10*

**Personal fitness evaluation,** *79*

**Personal fitness &**
**monitoring test,** *79*

**Pilates:**
*exercise equipment, 64*
*workout, 64*

**Plank:**
*side, 151*
*with leg extension, 149*

**Processed foods,** *159*

**Public transportation,** *30, 32*

**Push-up side plank combo,** *151*

**Push-ups:**
*assisted, 45*
*diamond, 123*
*modified, 101*
*modified-wide, 118*
*plyometric, 139*

**Posture:**
*erect, 7*
*maintain, 9*
*poor, 33*
*proper, 33*
*upright, 119*

**Progressive Exerciser,** *18, 86,*
*89, 91-92, 100, 188*

## Q

**Questionnaire,** *exercise, 67-68*

## R

**Rate of perceived exertion,** *195*

**Recipes:**
*beef and cabbage bake, 169*
*cannelloni with mushrooms, 176*
*cheese and onion quiche, 180*
*cheese stuffed zucchini, 179*
*chicken and bean stir fry, 172*
*chili omelet, 178*
*coriander beef stew, 171*
*coriander turkey burgers, 174*
*garlic & mushroom pasta, 175*
*gingerbread chicken kebabs, 173*
*ham and mushroom*
*cannelloni, 177*
*meatballs in tomato sauce, 170*

**Repetitions,** *13-15, 43-47, 79,*
*92-93, 99-100, 109, 112, 117, 121-*
*125, 128, 132, 136, 138, 140-141,*
*143, 145-146, 185, 197*